Diagnosis in Acute Medicine

Sherif
BM B

Specialty Registrar in Respiratory Medicine
East Midlands Deanery

Foreword by
Ian Pavord
DM FRCP
Consultant Physician and Honorary Professor of Medicine
Department of Respiratory Medicine, Thoracic Surgery and Allergy
University Hospitals of Leicester NHS Trust
Glenfield Hospital, Leicester

Radcliffe Publishing
Oxford • New York

Radcliffe Publishing Ltd
18 Marcham Road
Abingdon
Oxon OX14 1AA
United Kingdom

www.radcliffe-oxford.com

Electronic catalogue and worldwide online ordering facility.

British Library Cataloguing in Publication Data

A catalogue record for this book is available from the British Library.

ISBN-13: 978 184619 433 7

The paper used for the text pages of this book is FSC certified. FSC (The Forest Stewardship Council) is an international network to promote responsible management of the world's forests.

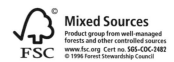

Mixed Sources
Product group from well-managed
forests and other controlled sources
www.fsc.org Cert no. SGS-COC-2482
© 1996 Forest Stewardship Council

FSC

Typeset by Phoenix Photosetting, Chatham, Kent
Printed and bound by TJI Digital, Padstow, Cornwall

Contents

Foreword   v

Preface   vi

About the author   vii

List of abbreviations   viii

Section 1: Introduction to medical diagnosis
  1   Information gathering and interpretation   1
  2   Diagnostic thinking   4

Section 2: Critical illness
  3   The critically ill patient   7
  4   Acute respiratory illness   10
  5   Shock   18
  6   Coma and reduced level of consciousness   22
  7   Acute kidney injury   27

Section 3: Cardiovascular and respiratory presentations
  8   Pleuritic chest pain   33
  9   Non-pleuritic chest pain   37
 10 Palpitation   41
 11 Oedema   45
 12 Limb pain   49

Section 4: Gastrointestinal presentations
 13 Abdominal pain   51
 14 Nausea and vomiting   57
 15 Gastrointestinal haemorrhage   62
 16 Dysphagia   65
 17 Diarrhoea   68
 18 Constipation   72
 19 Abdominal swelling   74
 20 Jaundice   77

Section 5: Neurological presentations
 21 Headache   83
 22 Transient loss of consciousness   88
 23 Focal neurological deficit   91
 24 Acute visual loss   98
 25 Vertigo   101

Section 6: Miscellaneous presentations

26	Frequency of micturition	103
27	Haematuria	107
28	Joint pain or swelling	110
29	Back pain	114
30	Pyrexia of unknown origin	119
31	Anaemia	124
32	Skin rash	129

Section 7: Biochemical abnormalities

33	Acid–base disturbances	133
34	Hyponatraemia	140
35	Hypernatraemia	144
36	Hypokalaemia	147
37	Hyperkalaemia	150
38	Hypocalcaemia	152
39	Hypercalcaemia	154

Index	157

Foreword

This book is aimed at medical students and junior doctors who would like to become excellent clinicians. What is it that sets apart the excellent clinician? Unfortunately, it is more than just mastery of facts and success in undergraduate and postgraduate examinations. Excellent clinicians have an instinct for the likely diagnosis every bit as sharp as the professional gambler's instinct for backing the right horse. This is honed by an extensive knowledge of the differential diagnosis and a forensic ability to determine the likely favourites and back markers. They are aware that odds may be altered by extraneous factors; they know which conditions are potentially disastrous and need to be actively ruled out. Once the correct diagnosis is made, excellent clinicians take decisive action.

This book is unique in that it addresses all these factors in relation to common symptom-based presentations. It provides an extensive list of potential causes of a wide variety of clinical presentations. Importantly, the common and important conditions are highlighted. This allows the clinician to begin to estimate the pre-test probability of different conditions, information that is essential to correctly interpret the results of clinical examinations and further investigations. The first two chapters are an excellent introduction to the diagnostic process. I recommend that they are read carefully.

Patients are rather more interested in treatments than in diagnostic labels, and it is important to remember that the diagnosis is only a stepping point on the way to treatment and prognostic decisions. The book emphasises the basic principles of management; it does not attempt to deal with treatment of individual conditions or methods of appraising these treatments. However, junior clinicians who have a sound grasp of these principles will be in a strong position to study and evaluate more complex, disease-specific treatment protocols.

When asked about his obsessional practice regime, the professional golfer Gary Player likes to say 'The harder I practice, the luckier I get.' This maxim is as true in clinical practice as it is in golf. No book can replace hard work on the ward and in clinics, but books can speed up the acquisition of skills by fostering sound basic principles and developing the right instincts. *Diagnosis in Acute Medicine* is particularly helpful in this regard. I strongly recommend it.

Professor Ian Pavord
Consultant Physician and Honorary Professor of Medicine
Department of Respiratory Medicine
Glenfield Hospital, University Hospitals of Leicester NHS Trust
April 2010

Preface

Medical students and junior doctors have traditionally learned medicine disease by disease, and most medical textbooks are still organised in this way. However, more recently the tide has begun to turn towards a more symptom-based approach to learning clinical medicine. Many medical schools are embracing problem-based learning, and in the postgraduate field the *Curriculum for General Internal Medicine*, published by the Royal College of Physicians in 2009, specifies symptom-specific rather than disease-specific competencies to be obtained by doctors in training. However, it should not be supposed that medical students and junior doctors can dispense with the traditional body of knowledge comprising the epidemiology, aetiology, pathology and clinical features of each condition, as mastery of this knowledge is essential in order to apply the problem-based approach effectively.

The purpose of this book is to present a logical structured approach to the diagnosis and initial management of the acutely unwell adult. For each clinical presentation, the relevant pathophysiology is first discussed and a comprehensive table of differential diagnoses is provided, with common causes highlighted in bold type. Next, the generic emergency management of the clinical presentation is described, and important diagnoses that should not be missed are pointed out. Finally, the history, examination findings and investigations that are relevant to assessing the patient's condition or making the diagnosis are explained.

Readers of this book are encouraged to keep certain thoughts uppermost in their mind while engaged in the diagnostic process. First, diagnosis is always a means to an end, namely treatment, and never an end in itself. An investigation that will not contribute to a change in the patient's management should not be performed. Secondly, *common things are common*. Being able to suggest an uncommon and highly unlikely cause of a given symptom is neither useful to the patient nor impressive to examiners. In fact it requires far more skill and judgement to arrive at the *most likely* diagnosis for a given clinical scenario, bearing in mind that atypical presentations of common conditions occur far more often than typical presentations of rare conditions. Finally, the reader is encouraged to subject both their own and other people's initial impressions to critical analysis at every stage, as many errors are made due to failure to revise the initial diagnosis in the light of new evidence.

This book is aimed primarily at senior medical students as well as junior doctors in their first four years after qualifying. It is during this crucial period that doctors in training lay down the foundations of their clinical practice and hone the systems of diagnostic thought that will serve them throughout their careers. If this volume can help its readers to think logically and systematically about the clinical problems that they encounter in their practice, it will have achieved its aim.

Sherif Gonem
April 2010

About the author

Sherif Gonem BM BSc MRCP graduated from the University of Southampton in 2004 with a Bachelor of Medicine degree, having completed an intercalated Bachelor of Science degree with first class honours the previous year. He spent the first two years of his postgraduate training at Southampton General Hospital, and subsequently completed his core medical training at City Hospital, Birmingham and Queen Alexandra Hospital, Portsmouth. He passed the MRCP examination in July 2007 and was appointed to his current post as a Specialty Registrar in Respiratory Medicine in the East Midlands Deanery in August 2008. Sherif has a keen interest in teaching both medical students and junior doctors, and has taught on the Care of the Critically Ill Medical Patient (CRIMP) course, as well as organising and delivering a module on acute medicine for medical students at the University of Leicester.

List of abbreviations

5-HIAA	5-Hydroxyindoleacetic acid
A–a	Alveolar–arterial
AACG	Acute angle-closure glaucoma
ABG	Arterial blood gas
ACE	Angiotensin-converting enzyme
AChR	Acetylcholine receptor
ACTH	Adrenocorticotropic hormone
ADEM	Acute disseminated encephalomyelopathy
ADH	Antidiuretic hormone
AG	Anion gap
AIDS	Acquired immune deficiency syndrome
AILD	Angioimmunoblastic lymphadenopathy with dysproteinaemia
AKI	Acute kidney injury
ALP	Alkaline phosphatase
ALT	Alanine aminotransferase
AMA	Anti-mitochondrial antibody
ANA	Anti-nuclear antibody
ANCA	Anti-neutrophil cytoplasmic antibody
ANNA	Anti-neuronal nuclear antibody
APTR	Activated partial thromboplastin time
ARDS	Acute respiratory distress syndrome
AST	Aspartate aminotransferase
BCG	Bacillus Calmette-Guérin
BRBNS	Blue rubber bleb naevus syndrome
CADASIL	Cerebral autosomal dominant arteriopathy with subcortical infarcts and leukoencephalopathy
cANCA	Cytoplasmic anti-neutrophil cytoplasmic antibody
CANOMAD	Chronic ataxic neuropathy, ophthalmoplegia, M-protein, agglutination and disialosyl antibodies
CEA	Carcinoembryonic antigen
CIDP	Chronic inflammatory demyelinating polyneuropathy
CINCA	Chronic infantile neurological, cutaneous and articular syndrome
CK	Creatine kinase
CMV	Cytomegalovirus
CNS	Central nervous system
COHb	Carboxyhaemoglobin
COPD	Chronic obstructive pulmonary disease
CPAP	Continuous positive airway pressure
CPM	Central pontine myelinolysis
CRP	C-reactive protein
CSF	Cerebrospinal fluid
CT	Computed tomography
CTPA	Computed tomography pulmonary angiogram
CXR	Chest X-ray
dsDNA	Double-stranded deoxyribonucleic acid
DVLA	Driver and Vehicle Licensing Agency
EABV	Effective arterial blood volume
EBV	Epstein–Barr virus
ECG	Electrocardiogram
EEG	Electroencephalogram
ENA	Extractable nuclear antigens
ENT	Ear, nose and throat
ERCP	Endoscopic retrograde cholangiopancreatogram
ESR	Erythrocyte sedimentation rate
FBC	Full blood count
FiO_2	Fractional inspired oxygen concentration
FVC	Forced vital capacity

G6PD	Glucose-6-phosphate dehydrogenase
GAD	Glutamic acid decarboxylase
GBM	Glomerular basement membrane
GCS	Glasgow Coma Scale
GI	Gastrointestinal
GM-CSF	Granulocyte-macrophage colony-stimulating factor
GORD	Gastro-oesophageal reflux disease
GTN	Glyceryl trinitrate
HAE	Hereditary angioedema
HELLP	Haemolysis, elevated liver enzymes and low platelet count
HaNDL	Headache and neurological deficits with cerebrospinal fluid lymphocytosis
HIDS	Hyperimmunoglobulinaemia D and periodic fever syndrome
HIV	Human immunodeficiency virus
HLA	Human leukocyte antigen
HONK	Hyperosmolar non-ketotic state
HSV	Herpes simplex virus
HTLV	Human T-cell lymphotropic virus
HUS	Haemolytic uraemic syndrome
IBD	Inflammatory bowel disease
IM	Intramuscular
INR	International normalised ratio
IV	Intravenous
JVP	Jugular venous pressure
LDH	Lactate dehydrogenase
LEMS	Lambert–Eaton myasthenic syndrome
LFTs	Liver function tests
LKMA	Liver–kidney microsomal antibodies
MC&S	Microscopy, culture and sensitivities
MCV	Mean corpuscular volume
MDMA	3,4-Methylenedioxymethamphetamine
MELAS	Mitochondrial myopathy, encephalopathy, lactic acidosis and stroke
MERRF	Myoclonic epilepsy with ragged red fibres
MPTP	1-Methyl-4-phenyl-1,2,3,6-tetrahydropyridine
MR	Magnetic resonance
MRCP	Magnetic resonance cholangiopancreatogram
MRI	Magnetic resonance imaging
MuSK	Muscle-specific kinase
NPV	Negative predictive value
NRTI	Nucleoside reverse transcriptase inhibitor
NSAID	Non-steroidal anti-inflammatory drug
NSTEMI	Non-ST elevation myocardial infarction
OGD	Oesophagogastroduodenoscopy
OHSS	Ovarian hyperstimulation syndrome
$PaCO_2$ or PCO_2	Arterial partial pressure of carbon dioxide
$PACO_2$	Alveolar partial pressure of carbon dioxide
PACS	Picture archiving and communications system
pANCA	Perinuclear anti-neutrophil cytoplasmic antibody
PaO_2 or PO_2	Arterial partial pressure of oxygen
PAP	Positive airway pressure
PAPA	Pyogenic arthritis, pyoderma gangrenosum and acne
PAS	Periodic acid Schiff
PCI	Percutaneous coronary intervention
PCR	Polymerase chain reaction
PET	Positron emission tomography
PML	Progressive multifocal leukoencephalopathy
POEMS	Polyneuropathy, organomegaly, endocrinopathy, monoclonal gammopathy and skin changes
PPV	Positive predictive value
PRES	Posterior reversible encephalopathy syndrome
PSA	Prostate-specific antigen
PTH	Parathyroid hormone
PTHrP	Parathyroid hormone-related peptide

PUO	Pyrexia of unknown origin
RAS	Renin–angiotensin system
RhF	Rheumatoid factor
RNP	Ribonucleoprotein
RS3PE	Remitting seronegative symmetrical synovitis with pitting oedema
SAAG	Serum-ascites albumin gradient
SAPHO	Synovitis, acne, pustulosis, hyperostosis and osteitis
SARS	Severe acute respiratory syndrome
SBE	Standard base excess
SC	Subcutaneous
SeHCAT	^{75}Se-homocholic acid taurine
SIADH	Syndrome of inappropriate antidiuretic hormone secretion
SLE	Systemic lupus erythematosus
SMA	Smooth muscle antibody
SNS	Sympathetic nervous system
SSRI	Selective serotonin reuptake inhibitor
STEMI	ST elevation myocardial infarction
SUNA	Short-lasting, unilateral, neuralgiform headache attacks with cranial autonomic symptoms
SUNCT	Short-lasting, unilateral, neuralgiform headache attacks with conjunctival injection and tearing
SVC	Superior vena cava
TFTs	Thyroid function tests
TINU	Tubulointerstitial nephritis and uveitis
TPHA	*Treponema pallidum* haemagglutination test
TPO	Thyroid peroxidase
TRAPS	Tumour necrosis factor receptor-associated periodic fever syndrome
TTP	Thrombotic thrombocytopaenic purpura
U&Es	Urea and electrolytes
US	Ultrasound
USS	Ultrasound scan
VDRL	Venereal disease research laboratory test
VGKC	Voltage-gated potassium channel
VIP	Vasoactive intestinal peptide
VKH	Vogt–Koyanagi–Harada
VMA	Vanillylmandelic acid
V/Q	Ventilation/perfusion
VZV	Varicella zoster virus
WBC	White blood cell
α1-AT	α1-Antitrypsin
β-HCG	β-Human chorionic gonadotropin
γ-GT	γ-Glutamyltransferase

CHAPTER 1

Information gathering and interpretation

The process of diagnosis begins with eliciting the patient's presenting complaint; there are approximately 40 complaints that commonly present to general physicians. There then follows a process of information gathering, consisting of the history, examination and investigations. Either during or at the end of this phase, the information is synthesised, enabling a decision to be made as to the final diagnosis.

HISTORY
The history is the most important part of the clinical evaluation. Most studies have found that approximately 80% of diagnoses are made from the history, 10% from the examination and 10% from investigations.[1] The information elicited from the history may be divided into two main categories. First, the presenting complaint and the history of the presenting complaint provide the story of the patient's illness, sometimes known as the 'illness script' Secondly, the personal details, past medical history, drug history, family history and social history provide the context in which the illness script may be interpreted. This is why senior clinicians who are presenting a case to a colleague will often begin with a few salient points from the past medical history or even the social history before describing the presenting complaint, and will prefer cases to be presented to them in this way.

EXAMINATION
In most cases, the history should allow a differential diagnosis – that is, a series of diagnostic hypotheses – to be formed. The primary aim of the physical examination is to test these hypotheses, looking specifically for evidence for and against each one. However, it is also desirable that a complete screening physical examination of all systems be carried out in each patient, first in order to detect unsuspected clinical signs that may be relevant to the presenting complaint, and secondly as a quick and easy screening tool for other pathology that may be unrelated to the current presentation.

INVESTIGATIONS
Investigations should be chosen in order to discriminate between the remaining diagnostic hypotheses following the history and examination. For instance, an ultrasound scan of the abdomen would be a useful investigation to distinguish between acute appendicitis and a ruptured ectopic pregnancy in a young woman with abdominal pain. However, an abdominal X-ray would be less useful, as it may be normal in both cases. The results of investigations should always be interpreted in light of the pre-test probability of the condition in question. For instance, a young healthy man with normal renal function has a low pre-test probability of having hyperkalaemia (a high serum potassium level). Thus, if a blood test unexpectedly shows this abnormality, it is more likely to represent a false positive than a true positive result, possibly due to haemolysis of the blood before analysis. The correct course of action in this case would be to repeat the test urgently.

INTERPRETATION OF TEST RESULTS
The purpose of diagnostic tests is to provide information that makes a given diagnosis either more or less likely. The probability of the diagnosis before the test is carried out is known as the pre-test probability, while

the probability of the diagnosis taking into account the test result is the post-test probability. The usefulness of a test for diagnosing any given condition may be described by two attributes of the test, namely its sensitivity and specificity. Importantly, these attributes are independent of the pre-test probability of the condition in the patient under investigation.

The sensitivity (Sn) of a test is the probability that a person with the diagnosis will have a positive test result. Thus a highly sensitive test is one that comes back positive in the vast majority of people with the diagnosis. Highly sensitive tests are good at ruling out diagnoses if they come back negative, but may be less informative if they are positive.

The specificity (Sp) of a test is the probability that a person without the diagnosis will have a negative test result. Thus a highly specific test is one that very rarely comes back positive in people without the diagnosis. Highly specific tests provide strong evidence for a diagnosis when positive, but may be less useful when they are negative.

The ideal diagnostic test would have a sensitivity and specificity of 100%. However, in practice, tests with high sensitivities often have less impressive specificities, and vice versa.

The positive predictive value (PPV) of a test is the probability that a patient with a positive test result in fact has the diagnosis in question. Similarly, the negative predictive value (NPV) of a test is the probability that a patient with a negative test result truly does not have the diagnosis in question.

The post-test probability of the diagnosis is therefore equal to:
➤ PPV in the case of a positive test
➤ (1 – NPV) in the case of a negative test.

Crucially, the positive and negative predictive values are highly dependent on the pre-test probability of the diagnosis. As discussed in the next chapter, there is a common tendency among all people, including doctors, to underestimate the importance of the pre-test probability and to overestimate the importance of the sensitivity and specificity of the test when interpreting test results (i.e. when estimating post-test probabilities).

For example, consider a 40-year-old man who presents with pleuritic chest pain. The admitting doctor estimates that the pre-test probability that this patient has a pulmonary embolism is 10%. She decides to perform a D-dimer blood test. Let us assume that the D-dimer has a sensitivity of 95% and a specificity of 60% for the diagnosis of pulmonary embolism. What is the post-test probability of pulmonary embolism if the D-dimer is positive? And what is it if the D-dimer is negative?

To answer these questions, we may draw a 2 × 2 contingency table, as shown in Figure 1.1, in which each box contains the probability of each contingency – for instance, a true positive or a false negative. The four probabilities should total one.

Each of the four boxes in the contingency table may be completed as follows (pre-test probability is represented by P):

$$\text{True positive (TP)} = P \times \text{Sn} \tag{1}$$
$$\text{False negative (FN)} = P \times (1 - \text{Sn}) \tag{2}$$
$$\text{True negative (TN)} = (1 - P) \times \text{Sp} \tag{3}$$
$$\text{False positive (FP)} = (1 - P) \times (1 - \text{Sp}). \tag{4}$$

Take a moment to convince yourself of the validity of the above four equations, making use of the definitions of sensitivity and specificity given earlier.

In the case of the 40-year-old man mentioned above, these values will be as follows:

Diagnosis

		Positive	Negative
Test	Positive	True positive (TP)	False positive (FP)
	Negative	False negative (FN)	True negative (TN)

Figure 1.1 Contingency table for diagnostic tests.

$$TP = 0.1 \times 0.95 = 0.095$$
$$FN = 0.1 \times 0.05 = 0.005$$
$$TN = 0.9 \times 0.6 = 0.54$$
$$FP = 0.9 \times 0.4 = 0.36.$$

The PPV is the probability that a positive test is a true positive. Therefore:

$$PPV = TP/(TP + FP) \tag{5}$$
$$= 0.095/(0.095 + 0.36)$$
$$= 0.209.$$

The NPV is the probability that a negative test is a true negative. Therefore:

$$NPV = TN/(TN + FN) \tag{6}$$
$$= 0.54/(0.54 + 0.005)$$
$$= 0.991.$$

Thus, in the case of a positive D-dimer, the post-test probability of pulmonary embolism will be 0.209 (20.9%), whereas in the case of a negative D-dimer the post-test probability will be equal to 1 – NPV, which in this case is 1 – 0.991, i.e. 0.009 (0.9%).

Note that even in the case of a positive D-dimer, the probability that this patient has a pulmonary embolism would only be approximately 20%. The diagnosis would still be more likely to be false than true. This is because the pre-test probability of the diagnosis was low (10%) and the specificity of the test was relatively low (60%), which means that false positives were fairly likely to occur. However, as pulmonary embolism is such an important diagnosis to make, due to its high untreated mortality, the doctor in this case would be obliged to investigate the patient further and initiate presumptive treatment.

In the case of a negative D-dimer, the post-test probability would fall dramatically compared with the pre-test probability, to just 0.9%. In this case, the probability of pulmonary embolism is so low that no further investigation is justified.

Notice that in the example given, a negative result had a much more pronounced effect on the post-test probability than a positive result. This is because the D-dimer has a low specificity but a high sensitivity for pulmonary embolism, which means that a positive result increases the probability of a positive diagnosis to a lesser extent than a negative result decreases the probability. Thus the D-dimer is a good test for ruling out the diagnosis of pulmonary embolism in cases with a low pre-test probability. However, it cannot be used to make a firm positive diagnosis. Further investigations such as ventilation/perfusion scanning or CT pulmonary angiography are required for this purpose.

Equations (1) to (4), in combination with equations (5) and (6), can be used to derive the following general formulae for the PPV and NPV. Note that the post-test probability of a given diagnosis in the case of a positive test is given by the PPV, whereas the post-test probability of the diagnosis in the case of a negative test is given by one minus the NPV.

$$PPV = \frac{P \times Sn}{(P \times Sn) + (1 - P)(1 - Sp)}$$

$$NPV = \frac{(1 - P) \times Sp}{((1 - P) \times Sp) + (P \times (1 - Sn))}$$

REFERENCE
1   Orient JM. *Sapira's Art and Science of Bedside Diagnosis.* 3rd ed. Philadelphia, PA: Lippincott Williams & Wilkins; 2005. p. 47.

CHAPTER 2

Diagnostic thinking

DIAGNOSTIC STRATEGIES

There are three main strategies that may be used to pursue a diagnosis. All three may be useful, depending on the particular case in question and the level of experience of the clinician:

1 **Diagnosis by exhaustion** is the method most often used by beginners in the field of diagnosis. This involves first collecting all of the data that are likely to be useful, including a thorough history and examination, and often a raft of diagnostic tests. Following this, an exhaustive list of possible diagnoses is compiled. Beginners, such as junior medical students, should not be discouraged from using diagnosis by exhaustion initially, as it is the most thorough method of reaching a diagnosis and, as a result, diagnostic possibilities are less likely to be missed. However, it is wasteful of time and resources and is thus inappropriate for routine clinical practice. Therefore, once students have achieved a certain level of background knowledge, they should begin to graduate to the hypothetico-deductive method.
2 The **hypothetico-deductive method** is a more dynamic process in which the clinician evaluates the information that they are receiving from the history to form hypotheses about the likely diagnosis. The doctor then asks appropriate questions, performs a focused clinical examination and requests the relevant investigations in order to test these hypotheses. During this process, the doctor has in their mind a short-list of possible diagnoses, weighted towards common, treatable and serious conditions. It is quite possible for one condition to drop off the list and another completely new diagnosis to be added to the list based on the history, examination and investigation findings as they are elicited. The hypothetico-deductive method is more efficient than diagnosis by exhaustion, but requires a certain amount of background knowledge and experience if it is to be implemented effectively.
3 **Pattern recognition** is a largely effortless and subconscious process by which an experienced clinician compares a particular patient's clinical presentation with their own accumulated memory bank concerning previous patients whom they have seen or read about. A close match prompts the making of an intuitive diagnosis. Clearly, the accuracy of this method depends on having extensive previous clinical experience to draw upon, so beginners should be discouraged from attempting to make diagnoses in this way. Even experienced doctors will regularly revert to the hypothetico-deductive method if pattern recognition does not yield an obvious diagnosis, and will check their initial impressions with a focused examination and appropriate investigations.

THE PATHOLOGICAL SIEVE

When confronted with a patient in whom the diagnosis is not obvious, it is useful to consider in turn each of the main pathological processes that may be causing the disease, rather than focusing on individual diagnoses. This approach is known as the pathological sieve. One such pathological classification of human disease is as follows:

Vascular
Autoimmune and inflammatory
Psychological
Infectious
Degenerative

Structural
Congenital
Environmental
Neoplastic
Toxic, endocrine and metabolic

This may be remembered using the mnemonic 'vapid scent.'

DIAGNOSTIC ERROR

Diagnostic errors may be classified into four main categories:
1 system-related factors (e.g. lack of diagnostic-quality PACS viewers)
2 inadequate knowledge or skills (e.g. failure to make a rare diagnosis due to unfamiliarity with the condition)

3   faulty data gathering (e.g. failure to perform an adequate physical examination)
4   cognitive errors.

COGNITIVE ERRORS IN DIAGNOSIS
No one – and this includes doctors – thinks in a purely logical fashion. Instead, they utilise various cognitive shortcuts, or heuristics, when solving clinical problems. These heuristics are common to all people, and lead to accurate solutions in most cases. However, in certain instances they may lead to cognitive biases that can result in diagnostic errors.

Cognitive biases that may result in diagnostic errors may be classified into three main groups, each of which is summarised below.

Faulty triggering and related errors
➤   Faulty triggering is a failure to consider the correct diagnosis in a patient whose presentation should prompt consideration of that diagnosis. For instance, a man of Indian origin presenting with a subacute history of cough, fever, night sweats and weight loss should prompt consideration of tuberculosis. If this diagnosis is not triggered in the clinician's mind, this may lead to the patient being misdiagnosed with a community-acquired pneumonia.
➤   Availability bias is a tendency to consider diagnoses that come more easily to mind to be more likely than others. Thus a doctor who has recently seen a case of aortic dissection may over-diagnose this condition in subsequent patients who present with chest pain.

Premature closure and related errors
➤   Premature closure is a failure to consider the possibility of alternative diagnoses once an initial diagnosis has been reached.
➤   The bandwagon effect is a tendency to accept uncritically a diagnostic label that has been applied to a patient by another clinician.
➤   Confirmation bias is the tendency to search for evidence to support the doctor's existing belief about the diagnosis, while dismissing or diminishing the importance of evidence against this diagnosis.

Failure to correctly evaluate probabilities
➤   Faulty context generation is the inaccurate estimation of a particular patient's pre-test probability of having a particular condition. For example, a 60-year-old man with chest pain should be regarded as having a higher pre-test probability of suffering from a myocardial infarction than a 20-year-old woman with similar symptoms.
➤   Base rate neglect, which is an extremely common cognitive error, is failure to take into account the pre-test probability of a particular condition when interpreting a clinical finding or investigation result. This results in overestimation of the significance of a positive test result when the pre-test probability of the condition in question is very low, or conversely, overestimation of the significance of a negative test result when the pre-test probability of the condition in question is very high.
➤   Faulty data interpretation is the overestimation or underestimation of the relevance of a particular clinical finding to the probability of the diagnosis in question.

The heuristics, or mental shortcuts, that all human beings use to solve day-to-day problems are clearly present for a good reason – they allow rough-and-ready solutions to complex problems to be found quickly. On the whole these heuristics work well, and for this reason they should not be abandoned altogether. However, by following a few simple rules it is possible to minimise their potential to induce diagnostic errors.
1   Systematically list the most likely and the most serious possible diagnoses for each patient at an early stage. Be comprehensive, but remember that 'Common things are common', or as they say in the USA, 'When you hear hoof-beats look for horses, not zebras.'
2   Be cautious about coming to a diagnosis too early, or uncritically accepting a diagnostic label that has already been assigned to a patient. Consider whether there are any other alternatives that fit the facts, and look for ways to distinguish between them. If new information comes to light that does not fit with the provisional diagnosis, or if the patient does not respond to treatment, challenge your initial assumptions.
3   Always take into account the pre-test probability of a diagnosis when interpreting a test result. Remember that no clinical finding or investigation result is entirely reliable. Get into the habit of starting with the pre-test probability and estimating how the test result will slide the probability up or down from there, rather than simply focusing on the test result in isolation. Better still, make use of a quantitative method, such as the formulae for positive and negative predictive values given above.

DIAGNOSIS IN CLINICAL PRACTICE
In general, diagnosis should be viewed as a means to an end, namely treatment, not as an end in itself. There are some cases in which a diagnosis need not be pursued any further, as it will not change the patient's management. For instance, consider the case of an elderly nursing home resident who is found to have iron-

deficiency anaemia. The causes of iron-deficiency anaemia include gastric or colonic cancer. However, if it is judged that the patient would not be fit for surgical intervention or chemotherapy even if a malignancy was to be discovered, there is no purpose in performing invasive tests such as colonoscopy or gastroscopy, as they would not change the patient's treatment. The correct course of action would be to treat the patient symptomatically with oral iron supplements. In other cases, the diagnostic process should be pursued partially, in order to rule out serious pathology, but not necessarily completed. For instance, chest pain is a very common emergency presentation, which has a number of serious causes and many less serious causes. Doctors who are managing a patient with acute chest pain should focus initially on diagnosing or ruling out serious pathology that requires urgent treatment, such as myocardial infarction, pulmonary embolism or aortic dissection, even if these diagnoses are not the most likely ones. Once this has been done, there is little benefit in distinguishing between the remaining possible causes, such as costochondritis or viral pleurisy, as they will each be treated similarly, with simple analgesia.

Remember that every investigation has a cost in terms of time, resources, patient discomfort and risk of complications. Before requesting any investigation, consider how the result may change the patient's management, and whether such a change is likely to significantly affect the patient's outcome. Weigh up whether these potential benefits outweigh the drawbacks of performing the investigation.

CHAPTER 3

The critically ill patient

In general, the management of any patient follows the familiar pattern of history, examination, investigations and finally treatment. However, this process takes time, and therefore a different approach is needed for the critically ill patient, for whom treatment is so urgent that it must be initiated before the diagnostic process has been fully completed. The most urgent clinical presentation of all is cardiorespiratory arrest (cardiac arrest). This is a clinical syndrome characterised by the absence of measurable cardiac output or adequate spontaneous respiratory effort. The standard algorithm for the management of cardiac arrest in the UK is published by the Resuscitation Council (UK),[1] and is shown in Figure 3.1. Advanced cardiac resuscitation is a practical skill that is best learned on dedicated courses. Regular refresher courses are mandatory to prevent de-skilling.

The following well-known schema is used to systematically assess and treat the critically ill patient. It is good practice to run through this schema with any acutely unwell patient before sitting down to take the history, to ensure that urgent treatment is not required:

➤ A – airway
➤ B – breathing
➤ C – circulation
➤ D – disability.

Throughout this book, in order to avoid repetition, it will be assumed that *airway, breathing and circulation have been secured before moving on to the next stage of management.* Chapters 4 and 5 describe in detail the assessment and management of the hypoxic patient and the shocked patient, respectively.

AIRWAY

Assessment
➤ Talk to the patient. If they can reply comfortably in full sentences, the airway is likely to be secure.
➤ Stridor, gurgling or snoring sounds are signs that the airway may be at risk.
➤ Patients with a reduced level of consciousness may be unable to protect their airway. Anyone with a Glasgow Coma Scale (GCS) score of 8 or less should be assumed to have an unprotected airway.
➤ Complete airway obstruction causes 'see-saw' breathing, in which the chest moves in as the abdomen moves out, and vice versa.

Treatment
➤ Open the mouth and use suction to remove any blood, vomitus or secretions. An unconscious patient who has vomited should be placed in the left lateral position, to prevent aspiration of vomitus.
➤ Open the airway by placing the patient in the 'sniffing the morning air' position, with the neck flexed and the head extended. The neck should not be manipulated if injury to the cervical spine is a possibility. In this instance, the airway may be opened by performing a jaw thrust, in which the mandible is pushed forward, thus lifting the tongue away from the posterior wall of the pharynx.
➤ Utilise airway adjuncts such as nasopharyngeal or oropharyngeal airways in order to maintain a patent airway. Note that these adjuncts will not protect against aspiration, and they will only be tolerated by patients with a reduced level of consciousness.

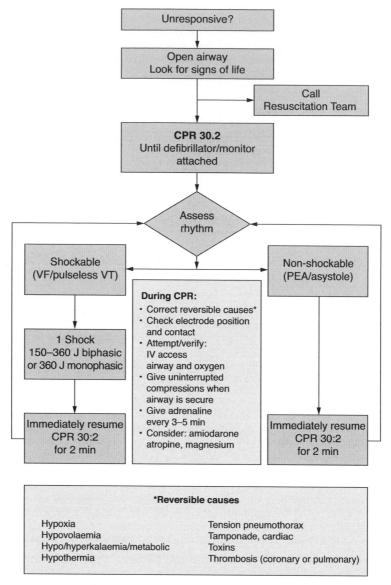

Figure 3.1 Algorithm for the management of cardiorespiratory arrest. Reproduced with kind permission of the Resuscitation Council (UK).

➤ Endotracheal intubation is the only way to completely secure the airway. Insertion of a laryngeal mask airway requires less skill and training and will allow the patient to be ventilated, but will not completely protect against aspiration.

BREATHING

Assessment

➤ Count the respiratory rate and assess the work of breathing and the use of accessory muscles of respiration. Observe the symmetry or otherwise of chest wall movement.
➤ Check the oxygen saturations with a pulse oximeter.
➤ Assess the tracheal position.
➤ Percuss and auscultate the chest, in particular checking for causes of respiratory compromise that require urgent treatment, such as tension pneumothorax and pulmonary oedema.

Treatment
➤ Provide oxygen. Most critically ill patients should initially be given high-flow oxygen via a reservoir bag mask, in order to maintain oxygen saturations of 94–98%.[2] Patients who are at risk of carbon dioxide retention, such as those with a history of chronic obstructive pulmonary disease (COPD), should receive controlled oxygen via a Venturi mask. The inspired oxygen concentration should be titrated to maintain the patient's oxygen saturation at between 88% and 92%.
➤ Perform an arterial blood gas analysis to assess the response to therapy.
➤ A patient who is hypoxic despite a high inspired oxygen concentration, or who has a respiratory acidosis, may require non-invasive or invasive respiratory support.
➤ Diagnose and treat the underlying cause (*see* Chapter 4).

CIRCULATION

Assessment
➤ Check the pulse and blood pressure.
➤ Check for signs of poor tissue perfusion (prolonged capillary refill time, weak thready pulse, confusion, reduced urine output).

Treatment
➤ Unless the patient is clearly fluid overloaded, provide an intravenous fluid challenge consisting of 250–500 ml of normal saline or colloid, and assess the response. This should be repeated until the patient is euvolaemic. Ruptured abdominal aortic aneurysm is one situation in which a degree of hypotension should be tolerated in order to prevent disruption of a partially formed thrombus and catastrophic haemorrhage.
➤ In difficult cases, consider central venous pressure monitoring in order to guide fluid resuscitation. In most cases, clinical assessment will suffice.
➤ If shock does not resolve following adequate fluid resuscitation, inotropic or vasopressor support may be required in an intensive-care setting.
➤ Diagnose and treat the underlying cause (*see* Chapter 5).

DISABILITY

Assessment
➤ Check the level of consciousness using the Glasgow Coma Scale (GCS).
➤ Check the capillary blood glucose concentration in any patient with a reduced level of consciousness.

Treatment
➤ Severe hypoglycaemia that is causing a reduced level of consciousness should be treated with IV glucose, for instance 25 ml of 50% glucose. This should be administered into a large vein and followed with a saline flush to reduce the risk of extravasation injury or phlebitis. Glucose-containing gels may be applied to the mucous membranes of the mouth as an interim measure while IV access is obtained.
➤ The assessment and management of the unconscious patient is described further in Chapter 6.

REFERENCES

1   Resuscitation Council (UK). *Resuscitation Guidelines 2005*. London: Resuscitation Council (UK); 2005.
2   O'Driscoll BR, Howard LS, Davison AG. BTS guideline for emergency oxygen use in adult patients. *Thorax*. 2008; **63** (Suppl. VI): vi1–68.

CHAPTER 4

Acute respiratory illness

PATHOPHYSIOLOGY AND AETIOLOGY

Acute respiratory illness may be defined as 'acute onset or worsening of any combination of respiratory failure, dyspnoea and cough.' It is among the most common reasons for admission to acute medical services, and patients presenting in this way are often critically ill. This chapter will discuss respiratory failure, dyspnoea and cough in an integrated fashion, as their causes overlap considerably. However, as discussed below, there are a number of important non-respiratory causes of dyspnoea and cough.

Respiratory failure may be defined as failure of the respiratory system to adequately oxygenate the blood or eliminate carbon dioxide, or both. Type 1 (hypoxaemic) respiratory failure is defined as an arterial partial pressure of oxygen (PaO_2) of less than 8 kPa while breathing room air, whereas type 2 (hypercapnic) respiratory failure is defined as an arterial partial pressure of carbon dioxide ($PaCO_2$) of greater than 6 kPa.

Respiratory function depends on two separate and independent processes, namely ventilation and gas exchange. Ventilation is the process whereby oxygen-rich ambient air is drawn into the alveoli during inspiration, and carbon-dioxide-laden alveolar gas is expelled during expiration. Gas exchange is the process whereby oxygen crosses from the alveolar gas to the pulmonary capillary blood, while carbon dioxide passes from the pulmonary capillary blood to the alveolar gas.

Gas exchange may be impaired by three mechanisms:

1 **Ventilation–perfusion mismatch (V/Q mismatch).** Optimum gas exchange occurs if ventilation and perfusion are closely matched throughout the lungs. V/Q mismatch results from perfusion of under-ventilated lung units or ventilation of under-perfused lung units. For instance, lung collapse or consolidation results in areas of lung being perfused but not adequately ventilated. This causes relatively deoxygenated blood to reach the systemic circulation, resulting in hypoxaemia.
2 **Shunt.** This is a special case of V/Q mismatch in which the V/Q ratio is 0. In other words, blood passes directly from the pulmonary to the systemic circulation without being oxygenated at all. Examples of this include intra-pulmonary arteriovenous malformations and cardiac defects such as ventricular septal defect with a right-to-left shunt.
3 **Impaired diffusion.** This is a failure of pulmonary capillary blood to fully equilibrate with alveolar gas during its transit through the lung. Impaired diffusion may be caused by processes such as interstitial lung disease that increase the distance that oxygen must travel in order to diffuse between the alveoli and capillaries.

Gas exchange abnormalities primarily affect oxygenation and result in type 1 respiratory failure. However, as long as alveolar ventilation can be increased to compensate, hypercapnia does not occur. This is because if ventilation of the normal alveoli is increased, extra carbon dioxide can be eliminated to compensate for the lack of effective gas exchange in the abnormal alveoli. However, hypoxaemia cannot be corrected in the same way because haemoglobin cannot be more than 100% saturated with oxygen, so there is an effective limit on the oxygen-carrying capacity of blood. This means that increasing ventilation in the normal alveoli cannot compensate for gas exchange abnormalities in the abnormal alveoli.

Alveolar ventilation may be impaired by dysfunction of any one of the links in the chain between the respiratory centre in the medulla and the lungs. The following mechanisms may result in ventilatory failure:

➤ respiratory centre depression
➤ high spinal cord injury
➤ peripheral neuropathy
➤ neuromuscular junction dysfunction
➤ respiratory muscle weakness
➤ chest wall deformity
➤ airway dysfunction
➤ reduced lung compliance.

Reduced alveolar ventilation impairs both the elimination of carbon dioxide and the uptake of oxygen, thus resulting in type 2 respiratory failure. A raised $PaCO_2$ is always the result of alveolar hypoventilation, except if the patient is actively re-breathing carbon dioxide (e.g. out of a brown paper bag).

The causes of type 1 and type 2 respiratory failure are listed in Table 4.1, with common causes highlighted in bold type.

Dyspnoea, or shortness of breath, may be defined as an abnormal awareness of breathing. Unlike sensations such as pain or light touch, the pathogenesis of dyspnoea is complex and incompletely understood; there is no specific 'shortness of breath receptor.' Dyspnoea most probably arises from a combination of various

Table 4.1 Causes of respiratory failure

Type 1 respiratory failure

Acute respiratory distress syndrome

Pulmonary oedema

Aspiration pneumonitis

Airway disease
- ▲ COPD
- ▲ Asthma
- ▲ Obstructive sleep apnoea
- ▲ Bronchiectasis
- ▲ Bronchiolitis

Bacterial infection
- ▲ Pneumonia
- ▲ Tuberculosis
- ▲ Atypical mycobacteria
- ▲ Lemierre's syndrome

Viral infection
- ▲ Influenza
- ▲ Parainfluenza
- ▲ Respiratory syncitial virus
- ▲ Adenovirus
- ▲ Varicella
- ▲ Cytomegalovirus
- ▲ SARS
- ▲ Hantavirus
- ▲ Miscellaneous

Miscellaneous infection
- ▲ *Pneumocystis jiroveci* pneumonia

Neoplasia
- ▲ Lung cancer
- ▲ Malignant mesothelioma
- ▲ Lymphangitis carcinomatosa
- ▲ Pulmonary lymphoma
- ▲ Lymphomatoid granulomatosis
- ▲ Epithelioid haemangio-endothelioma
- ▲ Pulmonary capillary haemangiomatosis

Idiopathic interstitial pneumonies
- ▲ Idiopathic pulmonary fibrosis
- ▲ Non-specific interstitial pneumonia
- ▲ Acute interstitial pneumonia
- ▲ Desquamative interstitial pneumonia
- ▲ Respiratory bronchiolitis-associated interstitial lung disease
- ▲ Lymphoid interstitial pneumonia
- ▲ Cryptogenic organising pneumonia

Occupational lung disease
- ▲ Asbestosis
- ▲ Coal-worker's pneumoconiosis
- ▲ Silicosis
- ▲ Berylliosis
- ▲ Miscellaneous

Eosinophilic lung disease
- ▲ Allergic bronchopulmonary aspergillosis
- ▲ Acute eosinophilic pneumonia
- ▲ Chronic eosinophilic pneumonia
- ▲ Hypereosinophilic syndrome
- ▲ Tropical pulmonary eosinophilia
- ▲ Löffler's syndrome
- ▲ Eosinophilia-myalgia syndrome

Gastrointestinal disease with pulmonary involvement
- ▲ Inflammatory bowel disease
- ▲ Coeliac disease
- ▲ Primary biliary cirrhosis

Complications of lung transplantation
- ▲ Primary graft dysfunction
- ▲ Acute rejection
- ▲ Chronic rejection

Complications of haematopoietic stem cell transplantation
- ▲ Diffuse alveolar haemorrhage
- ▲ Idiopathic pneumonia syndrome
- ▲ Engraftment syndrome
- ▲ Bronchiolitis obliterans

Inherited disease
- ▲ Hermansky–Pudlak syndrome

Type 2 respiratory failure

Airway disease
- ▲ COPD
- ▲ Asthma
- ▲ Obstructive sleep apnoea

Upper airway obstruction
- ▲ Anaphylaxis
- ▲ Angioedema
- ▲ Mastocytosis
- ▲ Epiglottitis
- ▲ Diphtheria
- ▲ Inhaled foreign body
- ▲ Tracheal stenosis
- ▲ Tumour
- ▲ Vocal cord paralysis or dysfunction
- ▲ Extrinsic compression

Chest wall and pleural disease
- ▲ Scoliosis/kyphoscoliosis
- ▲ Ankylosing spondylitis
- ▲ Chest trauma
- ▲ Thoracic surgery
- ▲ Diffuse pleural thickening
- ▲ Malignant mesothelioma

Reduced lung compliance
- ▲ Pulmonary oedema
- ▲ ARDS

Respiratory centre depression
- ▲ Obesity hypoventilation
- ▲ Central sleep apnoea
- ▲ Ethanol
- ▲ Benzodiazepines
- ▲ Opiates
- ▲ Barbiturates
- ▲ Brainstem damage
- ▲ Hypothyroidism
- ▲ Metabolic alkalosis

High cervical spinal cord injury

Peripheral neuropathy
- ▲ Guillain–Barré syndrome
- ▲ CIDP
- ▲ Motor neuron disease
- ▲ Multifocal motor neuropathy
- ▲ Charcot–Marie–Tooth disease
- ▲ Critical illness polyneuropathy
- ▲ Bilateral diaphragm paralysis
- ▲ Poliomyelitis
- ▲ Acute porphyria
- ▲ Miscellaneous

Neuromuscular junction blockade
- ▲ Myasthenia gravis
- ▲ LEMS
- ▲ Botulism
- ▲ Marine neurotoxins
- ▲ Tick paralysis
- ▲ Envenomation
- ▲ Organophosphates

Table 4.1 Causes of respiratory failure – *continued*

Type 1 respiratory failure

Fungal pneumonia
➤ Malarial lung
➤ Toxoplasmosis
➤ Helminth infection

Pleural disease
➤ **Pneumothorax**
➤ **Pleural effusion**
➤ **Empyema**
➤ **Haemothorax**

Pulmonary embolism
➤ **Venous thromboembolism**
➤ Chronic thromboembolic disease
➤ Tumour
➤ Amniotic fluid
➤ Fat
➤ Air

Right-to-left shunt
➤ Cyanotic congenital heart disease
➤ Pulmonary arteriovenous malformations
➤ Hepatopulmonary syndrome

Miscellaneous vascular disease
➤ Sickle-cell disease
➤ Hyperviscosity syndrome
➤ Primary pulmonary hypertension
➤ Pulmonary veno-occlusive disease
➤ Pulmonary vein stenosis

Drugs and toxins
➤ Amiodarone
➤ Bleomycin
➤ Methotrexate
➤ Busulphan
➤ Nitrofurantoin
➤ Paraquat
➤ Inhaled toxins
➤ Miscellaneous

Connective tissue disease
➤ Rheumatoid arthritis
➤ Systemic lupus erythematosus
➤ Systemic sclerosis
➤ Sjögren's syndrome
➤ Polymyositis
➤ Dermatomyositis
➤ Mixed connective tissue disease
➤ Ankylosing spondylitis

Vasculitis
➤ Wegener's granulomatosis
➤ Churg–Strauss syndrome
➤ Microscopic polyangiitis
➤ Goodpasture's disease
➤ Miscellaneous

➤ Gaucher's disease
➤ Neimann–Pick disease

Miscellaneous diffuse lung diseases
➤ **Sarcoidosis**
➤ **Hypersensitivity pneumonitis**
➤ Radiation pneumonitis
➤ Amyloidosis
➤ Pulmonary alveolar proteinosis
➤ Alveolar microlithiasis
➤ Langerhans cell histiocytosis
➤ Erdheim–Chester disease
➤ Lymphangioleiomyomatosis
➤ Lipoid pneumonia
➤ Idiopathic pulmonary haemosiderosis

Type 2 respiratory failure

Increased muscle tone
➤ Tetanus
➤ Strychnine poisoning
➤ Neuroleptic malignant syndrome
➤ Status dystonicus

Myopathy
➤ **Muscular dystrophy**
➤ Myotonic dystrophy
➤ Polymyositis
➤ Dermatomyositis
➤ Acid maltase deficiency
➤ Hypophosphataemia
➤ Miscellaneous

sensory inputs, including pulmonary stretch receptors, chest wall mechanoreceptors and central chemoreceptors, as well as a conscious awareness of the increased work of breathing.[1] There is a great deal of overlap between the causes of dyspnoea and respiratory failure, but it should be remembered that there are a number of important non-respiratory causes of dyspnoea, and conversely, not all causes of respiratory failure result in the sensation of dyspnoea. In particular, respiratory centre depression (e.g. due to opiate poisoning) causes type 2 respiratory failure without dyspnoea. The non-respiratory causes of dyspnoea are listed in Table 4.2, with common causes highlighted in bold type.

Table 4.2 Non-respiratory causes of dyspnoea

Cardiovascular	*Miscellaneous*
Congestive cardiac failure	Metabolic acidosis
Angina pectoris	Shock
Myocardial infarction	Sepsis
Cardiac arrhythmia	Reduced oxygen delivery
	➤ Anaemia
Cardiac tamponade	➤ Carbon monoxide poisoning
Acute valvular regurgitation	➤ Cyanide poisoning
	➤ Methaemoglobinaemia
Aortic dissection	➤ High altitude
Superior vena cava obstruction	Psychogenic
	➤ **Hyperventilation syndrome**
Cyanotic congenital heart disease	➤ **Panic attack**
	Miscellaneous
	➤ **Hyperthyroidism**
	➤ Gastro-oesophageal reflux disease

Coughing is a protective reflex characterised by the sudden forceful expulsion of air from the lungs, accompanied by the opening of an initially closed glottis. It results mainly from the stimulation of afferent mechanoreceptors and chemoreceptors in the upper airways and the large lower airways, to the level of the main bronchi. Stimuli arising from the nasal passages, sinuses and external ear may also result in cough. Efferent signals from the cough centre in the medulla cause the coordinated contraction of the respiratory musculature, resulting in sudden expulsion of air when the glottis opens. Cough is a non-specific feature of pulmonary disease, and may result from any of the causes of type 1 respiratory failure listed in Table 4.1. Extra-pulmonary causes of cough are listed in Table 4.3, with common causes highlighted in bold type.

EMERGENCY MANAGEMENT
➤ Assess the airway (*see* Chapter 3).
  - If there are signs of airway compromise such as stridor, arrange urgent anaesthetic input.
  - If impending upper airway obstruction is suspected, do not attempt to examine the throat without anaesthetic support, as complete airway occlusion may be precipitated.
  - Singed facial hair and soot in the nose or oropharynx are signs of significant smoke inhalation injury, and patients with these signs are at risk of airway oedema and compromise. Prophylactic endotracheal intubation should be considered early, as this may later become impossible due to the extent of airway oedema.
➤ Correct hypoxia with supplemental oxygen.
  - Oxygen may be delivered using devices that provide either a fixed flow of oxygen (nasal cannulae, simple face mask or reservoir bag mask) or a fixed fractional inspired oxygen concentration (FiO_2) (Venturi mask). Fixed flow devices do not provide a constant FiO_2, as the rate of oxygen delivery is fixed, and therefore if the respiratory minute volume increases, the FiO_2 will decrease, due to dilution of the inhaled oxygen with additional ambient air, and vice versa. Venturi masks are engineered to maintain a fixed FiO_2 regardless of the patient's minute volume and the flow of oxygen to the mask, provided it is above the minimum rate specified on the Venturi valve.
  - Most acutely hypoxic patients should be treated with a sufficient FiO_2 to maintain oxygen saturations of 94–98%.[2] However, a proportion of patients with chronic respiratory conditions such as COPD may develop hypercapnia when exposed to an excessively high FiO_2. In severe cases, this may lead to a downward spiral of narcosis and increasing respiratory depression. Thus patients who are

at risk of carbon dioxide retention should receive controlled oxygen therapy using a Venturi mask with the FiO_2 titrated to achieve oxygen saturations of approximately 88–92%. Each change in FiO_2 should be followed by an arterial blood gas 20–30 minutes later to ensure that the PaO_2 and $PaCO_2$ are acceptable.

- *Under no circumstances* should a patient be allowed to become hypoxaemic (saturations < 85%), due to concern about carbon dioxide retention. Hypoxia kills far more quickly than hypercapnia. A patient who is both hypoxaemic and hypercapnic is likely to be getting tired, and requires non-invasive or invasive respiratory support, **not** a reduction in FiO_2.

Table 4.3 Extra-pulmonary causes of cough

Upper airway	Miscellaneous
Rhinosinusitis	Gastro-oesophageal reflux disease
➤ Allergic	
➤ Viral	Pharyngeal pouch
➤ Bacterial	
➤ Fungal	ACE inhibitors
➤ Miscellaneous	
	External ear disorders
Laryngeal or tracheal infection	➤ Ear wax
➤ Croup	➤ Foreign body
➤ Influenza	
➤ Infectious mononucleosis	
➤ Measles	
➤ Bacterial tracheitis	
➤ Diphtheria	
➤ Pertussis	
➤ Miscellaneous	
Neoplasia	
➤ Pharyngeal	
➤ Laryngeal	
➤ Tracheal	
Extrinsic insults	
➤ Foreign body	
➤ Toxin inhalation	
Tracheal compression	
➤ Goitre	
➤ Aortic aneurysm	
➤ Vascular ring	
➤ Oesophageal tumour	
➤ Mediastinal mass	
➤ Miscellaneous	
Tracheal stenosis	
➤ Sarcoidosis	
➤ Amyloidosis	
➤ Relapsing polychondritis	
➤ Post-intubation	
➤ Trauma	
➤ Miscellaneous	
Structural tracheal abnormalities	
➤ Tracheomalacia	
➤ Tracheobronchomegaly	
➤ Tracheo-oesophageal fistula	
➤ Tracheopathia osteoplastica	
Lymphoid hypertrophy	
➤ Tonsilar	
➤ Adenoidal	
Vocal cord dysfunction	

➤ Perform a focused examination of the respiratory system, searching in particular for conditions that require immediate treatment.
  – Decompress a tension pneumothorax by inserting a 14-gauge cannula into the pleural space at the level of the second intercostal space in the mid-clavicular line.
  – Treat anaphylaxis with IM adrenaline (epinephrine), IV hydrocortisone and IV chlorphenamine, as well as IV fluid resuscitation.
  – Treat airflow limitation, as evidenced by wheeze or widespread reduced breath sounds, with nebulised (with or without IV) bronchodilators and oral (or IV) corticosteroids.
  – Treat pulmonary oedema with IV diuretics, and consider a GTN infusion or IV morphine.
  – Treat pneumonia with antibiotics according to local guidelines.
  – If opiate poisoning is suspected, give IV naloxone. Benzodiazepine overdoses may be treated with flumazenil, but not in a mixed overdose in which tricyclic antidepressants may have been taken, as in this case flumazenil may precipitate seizure.
➤ Provide respiratory support if required.
  – Failure to maintain an adequate PaO_2 despite a high FiO_2, or a persistent respiratory acidosis, indicates that non-invasive or invasive respiratory support is likely to be required. Non-invasive respiratory support involves the use of a tight-fitting mask that provides either a constant positive airway pressure (CPAP) throughout the respiratory cycle, or a variable positive airway pressure that is lower during expiration than during inspiration (bi-level PAP). Invasive respiratory support involves tracheal intubation and positive pressure ventilation.
  – There is convincing evidence that the early institution of bi-level PAP in patients with exacerbations of COPD and respiratory acidosis results in an improved outcome.[3] In addition, bi-level PAP is often effective in patients with type 2 respiratory failure due to other conditions, such as obstructive sleep apnoea, obesity hypoventilation and chest wall deformities. CPAP may be used to treat acute pulmonary oedema, as well as other causes of type 1 respiratory failure, although endotracheal intubation should not be delayed if a trial of non-invasive ventilation is unsuccessful. Certain conditions, such as life-threatening asthma, should be treated with intubation and invasive ventilation in the first instance if respiratory support is required.
➤ Massive haemoptysis is an uncommon but life-threatening emergency. Treatment is as follows.[4]
  – The patient should lie with the bleeding lung down to prevent blood entering the healthy lung. Intubation with a double-lumen endotracheal tube may be considered in order to isolate the bleeding lung.
  – Provide fluid resuscitation.
  – Nebulised adrenaline (epinephrine) (5–10 ml of 1:10 000) and oral tranexamic acid should be provided.
  – Bronchoscopy (preferably rigid) may be both diagnostic and therapeutic. Bleeding may be arrested by the use of balloon tamponade or the application of adrenaline (epinephrine) directly to the bleeding point.
  – Bronchial artery embolisation should be considered if available.
  – Surgical resection of the bleeding lobe may be performed as a last resort.

HISTORY
➤ The time course of the illness is a major diagnostic clue. For example, pneumothorax and pulmonary embolism may cause a sudden onset of dyspnoea, whereas pneumonia and exacerbations of COPD generally cause worsening dyspnoea over a period of hours to days.
➤ Exacerbating factors:
  – Orthopnoea, or dyspnoea that is worse in the supine position, is generally a symptom of pulmonary oedema, although it may also occur with emphysema, diaphragmatic paralysis and morbid obesity.
  – Trepopnoea is dyspnoea that is worse when lying on one side than on the other. Patients with unilateral lung disease tend to prefer to sleep with the normal lung down in order to maximise perfusion to this lung. Patients with congestive cardiac failure tend to prefer to sleep in the right lateral position.
  – Platypnoea is dyspnoea that is worse in the upright position. It occurs in the hepatopulmonary syndrome.
  – Dyspnoea that is worse at night may occur with pulmonary oedema, asthma or gastro-oesophageal reflux disease.
➤ Associated symptoms provide an important guide to the diagnosis.
  – Sputum production occurs with pulmonary infections, and with exacerbations of COPD, asthma or bronchiectasis.
  – Haemoptysis may occur with bronchiectasis, infection, malignancy, pulmonary embolism, pulmonary oedema, vasculitis or arteriovenous malformations.
  – Wheeze is caused by COPD, asthma or pulmonary oedema (so-called 'cardiac wheeze').
  – Stridor is a sign of upper airway obstruction, and urgent input from an anaesthetist is mandatory. Consider the possibility of anaphylaxis, especially if there is an urticarial rash.

- Pleuritic chest pain may occur with any pathology that causes pleural irritation (e.g. pneumonia or pulmonary embolism).
- Morning headaches and unrefreshing sleep are symptoms of obstructive sleep apnoea.
- Muscle pain or weakness may be a clue to neuromuscular disease.
- Sensory loss may occur with Guillain–Barré syndrome.

➤ Important features of the social history include a full occupational history, and details of current or previous smoking. Use of illicit drugs, particularly heroin, should be inquired about in the case of respiratory depression.

EXAMINATION

➤ Check for evidence of airway obstruction such as stridor.

➤ Check the vital signs (respiratory rate, pulse, blood pressure, temperature and oxygen saturations).

➤ Check the level of consciousness using the Glasgow Coma Scale (GCS). Hypoxia and hypercapnia may themselves cause a reduced level of consciousness if severe. Consider the possibility of poisoning with ethanol, opiates, benzodiazepines or barbiturates in patients with a low GCS, especially if the respiratory rate is low. Pinpoint pupils are a sign of opiate poisoning.

➤ Perform a general inspection. Increased work of breathing and use of accessory muscles of respiration suggests severe respiratory compromise. Prolonged expiratory phase or pursed lip breathing occurs with COPD. Obesity is a marker of possible obstructive sleep apnoea or obesity hypoventilation.

➤ Examine the hands. Check for a hypercapnic flap. Inspect for clubbing, which may be present with bronchiectasis, pulmonary fibrosis or lung cancer.

➤ Palpate the pulse, noting the rate, rhythm and character. A bounding pulse is a sign of hypercapnia.

➤ Assess the jugular venous pressure. It may be raised with massive pulmonary embolism, cor pulmonale or tension pneumothorax.

➤ Check for cervical or axillary lymphadenopathy, which may occur with metastatic malignancy.

➤ Check the tracheal position. Deviation away from the diseased lung occurs with a tension pneumothorax or large pleural effusion. Deviation towards the diseased lung occurs with pulmonary collapse or fibrosis.

➤ Inspect the chest for kyphosis, scoliosis, pectus carinatum or excavatum and the hyper-expanded 'barrel chest' of COPD.

➤ Assess chest expansion. This is reduced by lobar or lung collapse, pneumothorax or a large pleural effusion.

➤ Vocal fremitus and resonance are increased with consolidation and reduced with pneumothorax or pleural effusion.

➤ Percuss and auscultate the chest:
- Wheeze occurs with asthma, COPD and pulmonary oedema.
- Fine crackles occur with pulmonary oedema and interstitial lung disease.
- Coarse crackles occur with pneumonia and bronchiectasis.
- Bronchial breathing is a sign of collapse or consolidation.
- Reduced breath sounds with dullness to percussion suggest pleural effusion, pleural thickening or a raised hemi-diaphragm.
- Reduced breath sounds with hyper-resonance to percussion occur with pneumothorax.

➤ Muscle weakness or sensory loss suggests neuromuscular pathology.

INVESTIGATIONS

The following core investigations are commonly required:

➤ Arterial blood gas analyis.
- An arterial blood gas analysis provides information about both the oxygenation and acid–base status of the patient. Note that metabolic acidosis (e.g. due to diabetic ketoacidosis) may cause dyspnoea, as the compensatory hyperventilation increases the work of breathing. Metabolic acid–base disturbances are discussed further in Chapter 33.
- As mentioned above, respiratory function depends on two related but independent processes, namely ventilation and gas exchange. The $PaCO_2$ is inversely proportional to alveolar ventilation, and therefore a raised $PaCO_2$ is a good guide to the presence of alveolar hypoventilation. Assessment of gas exchange abnormalities is more complex, as the PaO_2 is affected by gas exchange abnormalities and alveolar ventilation, as well as the fractional inspired oxygen concentration (FiO_2). Fortunately, a method exists for factoring out the effect of both ventilatory abnormalities and the FiO_2. The alveolar–arterial gradient (A–a gradient) is the difference between the partial pressure of oxygen in the alveolar gas (PAO_2) and in the arterial blood (PaO_2). A small difference is normal, due to the minor degree of V/Q mismatch and shunting that occurs in normal individuals. However, an abnormally raised A–a gradient is strong evidence for a gas exchange abnormality. The A–a gradient (kPa) is given by the following formula:

$$\text{A–a gradient} = (95 \times FiO_2) - (PaCO_2/0.8) - PaO_2$$

– The normal range for the A–a gradient while breathing room air is < 2 kPa in young non-smokers and < 4.0 kPa in smokers or the elderly.[5] The A–a gradient increases in magnitude as the FiO_2 increases, in both normal individuals and those with gas exchange abnormalities.

➤ CXR:
  – A variety of pathologies may be visualised, including pneumonia, pulmonary oedema, alveolar haemorrhage, interstitial lung disease, pleural effusion and pneumothorax.
➤ Blood tests:
  – FBC. Anaemia may cause shortness of breath. A raised WBC suggests infection.
  – CRP. This is raised with infection.
  – U&Es. Combined pulmonary and renal dysfunction may be caused by pneumonia with severe sepsis, cardiac failure or systemic vasculitis.
  – D-dimer. This test should be performed if pulmonary embolism is suspected.
  – Glucose. This is raised with diabetic ketoacidosis, an important non-respiratory cause of dyspnoea.
➤ ECG:
  – Check in particular for cardiac arrhythmias and evidence of myocardial ischaemia.
➤ Urine dip:
  – Suspect diabetic ketoacidosis if this is positive for glucose and ketones, in conjunction with a metabolic acidosis on the arterial blood gas. Haematuria suggests a pulmonary–renal syndrome such as Goodpasture's disease or systemic vasculitis.

The following further investigations may be required:
➤ CT of the chest. This provides further information about the lung parenchyma and may reveal a mass lesion.
➤ CT pulmonary angiogram or V/Q scan. This is used to diagnose pulmonary embolism.
➤ Pulmonary function tests. These are not generally performed in the acute setting, but may be required later to help to determine the underlying chronic pulmonary condition.
➤ Echocardiogram. Impaired left ventricular function is seen with congestive cardiac failure.
➤ Blood tests:
  – Carboxyhaemoglobin. This should be performed urgently on arterial blood if carbon monoxide poisoning is a possibility.
  – Troponin. This is performed 12 hours after the onset of symptoms and is a marker of myocardial damage. It is raised following a myocardial infarction, but also with congestive cardiac failure, renal failure and severe sepsis.
  – TFTs. Hyperthyroidism is an occasional cause of dyspnoea, whereas hypothyroidism may cause type 2 respiratory failure.
  – Autoimmune and vasculitis screen. ANA and ENA (connective tissue disease), RhF (rheumatoid lung disease), ANCA (Churg–Strauss syndrome, Wegener's granulomatosis), anti-GBM antibody (Goodpasture's disease).
  – Serum ACE. This is raised with sarcoidosis.
  – HIV test. This should be performed if opportunistic infection is suspected.
    CMV serology and PCR.
➤ Sputum microscopy and culture.
➤ Thoracocentesis. Pleural fluid should be analysed for protein, LDH, microscopy, culture and cytology.
➤ Bronchoscopy with bronchoalveolar lavage. This is particularly useful in immunocompromised patients in order to diagnose opportunistic pathogens such as *Pneumocystis jirovecii*.

REFERENCES

1 Porter JC. Dyspnea. In: Albert RK, Spiro SG, Jett JR (eds) *Clinical Respiratory Medicine*. 3rd ed. Philadelphia, PA: Mosby; 2008. pp. 293–4.
2 O'Driscoll BR, Howard LS, Davison AG. BTS guideline for emergency oxygen use in adult patients. *Thorax*. 2008; **63 (Suppl. VI)**: vi1–68.
3 National Institute for Clinical Excellence. National clinical guideline on management of chronic obstructive pulmonary disease in adults in primary and secondary care. *Thorax*. 2004; **59 (Suppl. I)**: i131–56.
4 Chapman S, Robinson G, Stradling J et al. *Oxford Handbook of Respiratory Medicine*. 2nd ed. Oxford: Oxford University Press; 2009. p. 43.
5 Cooper N, Cramp P. *Essential Guide to Acute Care*. London: BMJ Books; 2003. p. 52.

CHAPTER 5

Shock

PATHOPHYSIOLOGY AND AETIOLOGY

Shock is a pathophysiological entity characterised by failure of the cardiovascular system to provide adequate tissue perfusion.

The causes of shock may be classified according to mechanism into the following four categories:

1 **Cardiogenic:** failure of the heart to produce sufficient forward flow of blood within the circulation, resulting in reduced tissue perfusion pressures. This is most commonly due to cardiac arrhythmias or myocardial infarction.
2 **Obstructive:** obstruction to blood flow within the great vessels, or obstructed ventricular filling. This has four major causes, namely pulmonary embolism, cardiac tamponade, tension pneumothorax and aortic dissection.
3 **Hypovolaemic:** reduced effective circulating volume, resulting in reduced preload and thus reduced cardiac output and tissue perfusion pressures. Acute haemorrhage is the most common cause in clinical practice.
4 **Distributive:** failure of normal vasomotor control, causing widespread inappropriate vasodilatation. This results in hypotension and shunting of blood through capillary beds without effective tissue perfusion. Distributive shock is mediated by the systemic release of pro-inflammatory cytokines in conditions such as sepsis, pancreatitis and anaphylaxis, resulting in increased capillary permeability and arteriolar vasodilatation. If it is not rapidly corrected, this process can culminate in multiple organ failure and death.

The causes of shock are listed in Table 5.1, with common causes highlighted in bold type.

EMERGENCY MANAGEMENT

➤ Ensure that the airway is patent.
➤ Correct hypoxia, if present, using supplemental oxygen.
➤ Establish large-bore intravenous access.
➤ Unless the patient is clearly fluid overloaded, provide a fluid challenge – for example, 250–500 ml of normal saline or colloid given over 5–10 minutes, and assess the response. Repeat until the patient is clinically euvolaemic, unless a leaking abdominal aortic aneurysm is suspected, in which case a degree of hypotension should be tolerated in order to prevent disruption of a partially formed thrombus.
➤ Perform a rapid but thorough examination, searching for reversible causes of shock that require urgent treatment.
   – Decompress a tension pneumothorax by inserting a 14-gauge cannula into the pleural space at the level of the second intercostal space in the mid-clavicular line.
   – Cardiac arrhythmias that are causing haemodynamic instability should be treated with DC cardioversion in the case of tachyarrhythmias, and IV atropine, possibly followed by temporary pacing, in the case of bradyarrhythmias (*see* Chapter 10).
   – Treat anaphylaxis with IM adrenaline (epinephrine), IV hydrocortisone and IV chlorphenamine, as well as IV fluid resuscitation.
   – Treat sepsis with broad-spectrum antibiotics that are tailored to the likely source, after drawing blood cultures.
   – The management of myocardial infarction is described in Chapter 9.
   – Cardiac tamponade is treated with urgent pericardiocentesis and insertion of a pericardial drain.
   – Massive pulmonary embolism that is causing haemodynamic compromise should be treated with thrombolysis if there are no contraindications.[1] This treatment may need to be instituted on clinical grounds alone, and a senior clinician should be involved in the decision to treat. An urgent bedside echocardiogram may be helpful for distinguishing massive pulmonary embolism from other causes of obstructive shock, such as cardiac tamponade.
   – Urgent surgical intervention may be required for a number of causes of shock, including type A aortic dissection, ruptured abdominal aortic aneurysm, acute valvular regurgitation, acute ventricular septum or wall rupture, ruptured ectopic pregnancy and perforated intra-abdominal viscus.

Table 5.1 Causes of shock

Cardiogenic	*Obstructive*	*Hypovolaemic*	*Distributive*
Cardiac arrhythmia	Pulmonary embolism	Haemorrhage	Systemic inflammatory response syndrome
		⮞ Gastrointestinal	
Reduced myocardial contractility	Cardiac tamponade	⮞ Abdominal aortic aneurysm	⮞ Sepsis
			⮞ Pancreatitis
⮞ Myocardial infarction	Tension pneumothorax	⮞ Ectopic pregnancy	⮞ Trauma
⮞ Myocarditis		⮞ Obstetric	⮞ Burns
⮞ Peripartum cardiomyopathy	Aortic dissection	⮞ Intra-abdominal	⮞ Surgery
⮞ Stress-induced cardiomyopathy	Atrial thrombus or tumour	⮞ Intra-thoracic	⮞ Toxic shock syndrome
⮞ Myxoedema coma		⮞ Musculoskeletal	⮞ Fulminant hepatic failure
⮞ Refeeding syndrome			
⮞ Beriberi		Gastrointestinal	Anaphylaxis or anaphylactoid reaction
⮞ Drugs and toxins		⮞ Diarrhoea	
⮞ Heat stroke		⮞ Vomiting	
		⮞ Excessive stoma output	Neurogenic shock
Structural heart disease		⮞ Enterocutaneous fistula	⮞ Head injury
⮞ Acute valvular regurgitation		⮞ Nasogastric drainage	⮞ Spinal cord injury
⮞ Ventricular septal rupture			
⮞ Ventricular wall rupture		Cutaneous	Miscellaneous
⮞ Myocardial contusion		⮞ Burns	⮞ Acute haemolytic transfusion reaction
		⮞ Excessive sweating	⮞ Thyroid storm
			⮞ Phaeochromocytoma
		Renal	⮞ Mastocytosis
		⮞ Polyuria	⮞ Heavy metal poisoning
		⮞ Adrenal insufficiency	⮞ Envenomation
			⮞ Systemic capillary leak syndrome
		Third space losses	
		⮞ Ileus	
		⮞ Bowel obstruction	
		⮞ Pancreatitis	

➤ Shocked patients are critically unwell and require monitoring in a high-care environment. Invasive cardiovascular monitoring using arterial and central venous catheters may be required. Consider inotropic and/or vasoconstrictor support if shock persists despite adequate fluid resuscitation. Patients with cardiogenic shock may require support with an intra-aortic balloon pump pending definitive treatment such as percutaneous coronary intervention (PCI).

HISTORY
➤ The presenting complaint may give a clue to the underlying diagnosis.
  - Fever suggests sepsis.
  - Chest pain may occur with myocardial infarction, aortic dissection, pulmonary embolism or tension pneumothorax.
  - Palpitation may be due to a cardiac arrhythmia.
  - Shortness of breath may occur with any cause of shock, but in particular suggests pulmonary embolism, tension pneumothorax, anaphylaxis or pneumonia with severe sepsis.
  - Abdominal pain should prompt consideration of a surgical emergency such as a perforated peptic ulcer. Ruptured abdominal aortic aneurysm may cause abdominal, loin or back pain.
  - Haematemesis, coffee-ground vomiting, rectal bleeding and melaena are features of gastrointestinal haemorrhage.
➤ Inquire about any serious comorbidities or recent surgery. A past medical history of ischaemic heart disease or abdominal aortic aneurysm is particularly relevant.

EXAMINATION
➤ Signs of shock include hypotension, tachycardia, tachypnoea, reduced urine output and confusion.
➤ Early distributive shock may be associated with warm peripheries and a bounding pulse. Other forms of shock are associated with cool peripheries, prolonged capillary refill time and a weak thready pulse. Dry mucous membranes and reduced skin turgor occur with hypovolaemia.
➤ Inspect the patient for anaemia, cyanosis, jaundice, skin rashes or evidence of trauma.
➤ Palpate the pulse, noting in particular any abnormally fast or slow rhythm. Check for radio-radial or radio-femoral delay, which is a feature of aortic dissection.
➤ Measure the blood pressure. A postural drop in blood pressure is a sensitive early sign of hypovolaemia, but should not be measured if a patient is already hypotensive. Significant blood pressure difference between the arms may occur with aortic dissection.
➤ If cardiac tamponade is a possibility, check for pulsus paradoxus, defined as a drop in the systolic blood pressure of more than 10 mmHg on inspiration. This can be measured with a normal sphygmomanometer, but the technique requires some practice.
➤ Assess the jugular venous pressure (JVP). Raised JVP is associated with cardiogenic or obstructive shock.
➤ Palpate the precordium for a right ventricular heave or a palpable pulmonary second heart sound. These are signs of pulmonary hypertension, and may occur with massive pulmonary embolism.
➤ Auscultate the heart.
  - Cardiac tamponade may be associated with quiet heart sounds.
  - Gallop rhythm with a third heart sound suggests cardiac failure.
  - A prominent pulmonary second heart sound may occur with massive pulmonary embolism.
  - Cardiac murmurs may be indicative of acute valvular regurgitation or ventricular septal rupture.
➤ Check the tracheal position. The trachea will be deviated away from the side of a tension pneumothorax.
➤ Percuss and auscultate the lung fields for evidence of tension pneumothorax, pneumonia or pulmonary oedema. The presence of pulmonary oedema suggests that the cause of shock is cardiogenic or obstructive.
➤ Check carefully for the presence of an abdominal aortic aneurysm, as well as for abdominal tenderness or peritonism.
➤ Perform a rectal examination to check for melaena or rectal bleeding.

INVESTIGATIONS
The following core investigations are commonly required:
➤ Blood tests:
  - FBC. Anaemia suggests haemorrhage, whereas a raised WBC is a feature of sepsis.
  - U&Es. Shock may be associated with acute kidney injury.
  - LFTs. Fulminant hepatic failure may be a cause or consequence of shock.
  - CRP. This is raised with sepsis.
  - TFT. Thyroid storm is a rare cause of shock.
  - Amylase. This is raised with pancreatitis.
  - Lactate. This is a marker of the severity of tissue hypoperfusion.
  - Clotting screen. This may be deranged due to liver dysfunction or disseminated intravascular coagulation, a possible feature of the systemic inflammatory response syndrome.
  - Group and save.

➤ Blood culture.
➤ ABG. This may reveal a metabolic acidosis due to the build-up of lactic acid produced by poorly perfused tissues.
➤ CXR. This may reveal pneumonia, pulmonary oedema or tension pneumothorax. A widened mediastinum suggests aortic dissection, whereas a globular heart suggests pericardial effusion. Subdiaphragmatic air is indicative of a perforated abdominal viscus.
➤ ECG. Cardiac arrhythmias, myocardial ischaemia or evidence of a pericardial effusion may be seen.
➤ Pregnancy test.

The following further investigations may be considered in certain cases:
➤ Echocardiogram. This may help to diagnose a number of cardiogenic or obstructive causes of shock. In particular, echocardiography may reveal ventricular wall motion abnormalities associated with myocardial ischaemia or dysfunction, cardiac tamponade, right ventricular strain associated with massive pulmonary embolism, acute valvular regurgitation or ventricular septal rupture.
➤ Gastroscopy or flexible sigmoidoscopy may be required to diagnose and/or treat acute gastrointestinal haemorrhage.
➤ Thoracic CT with contrast is used to diagnose a pulmonary embolism or aortic dissection.
➤ Abdominal imaging via US or CT scanning may reveal a leaking abdominal aortic aneurysm, ruptured ectopic pregnancy or other source of intra-abdominal haemorrhage. Evidence for other surgical emergencies, such as a perforated viscus or pancreatitis, may also be visualised.
➤ In cases of sepsis, further microbiological specimens may be required, such as cultures of sputum, urine, stool or cerebrospinal fluid.
➤ Short tetracosactide test is used to diagnose adrenal insufficiency.

REFERENCE
1   British Thoracic Society Standards of Care Committee Pulmonary Embolism Guideline Development Group. British Thoracic Society guidelines for the management of suspected acute pulmonary embolism. *Thorax*. 2003; **58**: 470–84.

CHAPTER 6

Coma and reduced level of consciousness

PATHOPHYSIOLOGY AND AETIOLOGY

Coma and reduced level of consciousness may result either from global cerebral dysfunction or from pathology affecting the reticular activating system (the 'on-off' switch of consciousness), located in the brainstem. Global cerebral dysfunction may be caused by systemic disease or by specific central nervous system disorders. On the other hand, damage to the reticular activating system may result from pathology directly affecting the brainstem, or from indirect compression of this area due to raised intracranial pressure. The mechanisms of coma and reduced conscious level may thus be summarised as follows:
➤ global cerebral dysfunction:
  – systemic pathology
  – central nervous system pathology
➤ reticular activating system damage:
  – local pathology
  – raised intracranial pressure.

In clinical practice, the causes of coma and reduced conscious level are most conveniently classified into systemic and central nervous system categories. Local central nervous system pathology may be further classified into infectious, inflammatory, vascular, neoplastic and miscellaneous categories. Table 6.1 lists the causes of coma and reduced level of consciousness, with common causes highlighted in bold type. Of note, confusion in the elderly may be precipitated by almost any acute illness. Conditions that commonly present with acute confusion in the elderly include urinary retention, constipation and myocardial infarction.

EMERGENCY MANAGEMENT

1 Ensure patency of the airway.
  ➤ Airway adjuncts such as Guedel or nasopharyngeal airways may be sufficient, but tracheal intubation is often required.
  ➤ In general, a patient with a GCS score of 8 or less is not considered capable of protecting their airway, and should be intubated.
2 Assess and treat respiratory and circulatory dysfunction in the normal way.
3 Treat the readily reversible causes of coma.
  ➤ Severe hypoglycaemia should be treated with IV glucose, for instance 25 ml of 50% glucose. This should be administered into a large vein and followed with a saline flush to reduce the risk of extravasation injury or phlebitis.
  ➤ If opiate poisoning is suspected, a trial of naloxone is indicated.
  ➤ Give IV thiamine if there is known or suspected alcohol dependency.
  ➤ If bacterial meningitis or viral encephalitis is suspected, give empirical IV antibiotics (according to local policy) or IV aciclovir, respectively.
4 Further management will depend on the underlying cause.

HISTORY

Collateral history, particularly from friends and relatives, work colleagues and ambulance personnel, is of vital importance. The following items of information should be elicited:
➤ time course of the illness
➤ associated symptoms, including fever, rash, headache, neck pain or stiffness, nausea or vomiting, focal weakness or sensory loss, vertigo, diplopia and jaundice
➤ evidence of drug overdose (e.g. empty packaging)
➤ past medical history
➤ allergies
➤ drug history
➤ illicit drug use

Table 6.1 Causes of coma or reduced level of consciousness

Systemic	Local	Vascular disease	Inflammation	Miscellaneous
Common causes of confusion in the elderly	**Infection**	Intracranial haemorrhage	Systemic lupus erythematosus	Head injury
➤ Urinary retention	Encephalitis	➤ Intracerebral	Sarcoidosis	Seizure disorders
➤ Constipation	➤ HSV 1 and 2	➤ Infratentorial	Aseptic meningitis	➤ **Status epilepticus**
➤ Myocardial infarction	➤ Herpes zoster virus	➤ Subarachnoid	Malignant meningitis	➤ **Post-ictal state**
➤ Pain	➤ Epstein–Barr virus	➤ Subdural	Autoimmune encephalopathy	➤ Temporal lobe epilepsy
	➤ Enteroviruses	➤ Extradural	➤ Limbic encephalitis	Neoplasia
Impaired oxygen delivery	➤ HIV		➤ Hashimoto's encephalopathy	➤ Primary brain tumour
➤ **Shock**	➤ Rabies	Cerebral or brainstem ischaemia	➤ Bickerstaff's encephalitis	➤ Brain metastasis
➤ **Hypoxia**	➤ West Nile virus	➤ **Thromboembolic stroke**		➤ Lymphoma
	➤ PML	➤ Pituitary apoplexy		➤ Bing–Neel syndrome
Endogenous toxins	➤ *Listeria monocytogenes*	➤ Cerebral venous thrombosis		Demyelination
➤ **Sepsis**	➤ Amoebic encephalitis	➤ Atrial myxoma		➤ Multiple sclerosis
➤ **Hypercapnia**	➤ Cerebral malaria	➤ Endocarditis		➤ Acute disseminated encephalomyelitis
➤ **Hepatic failure**	➤ African trypanosomiasis	➤ Decompression sickness		➤ Central pontine myelinolysis
➤ **Renal failure**	➤ Miscellaneous	➤ Carotid or vertebral artery dissection		➤ Marchiafava–Bignami disease
➤ Acute porphyria		➤ Basilar migraine		
➤ Ureterosigmoidostomy	Meningitis			Miscellaneous
➤ Multiple myeloma[1]	➤ **Viral**	CNS vasculopathy		➤ Hydrocephalus
	➤ **Bacterial**	➤ Vasculitis		➤ Subdural hygroma
Endocrine	➤ **Tuberculous**	➤ TTP/HUS		➤ MELAS
➤ **Hypoglycaemia**	➤ Fungal	➤ Antiphospholipid syndrome		➤ Radiation encephalopathy
➤ **Diabetic ketoacidosis**		➤ Sneddon's syndrome		➤ Catatonia
➤ **Hyperosmolar non-ketotic state**		➤ Cholesterol embolism		
➤ Thyroid storm		➤ Hyperviscosity syndrome		
➤ Myxoedema coma		➤ Intravascular lymphoma		
➤ Adrenal insufficiency		➤ Lymphomatoid granulomatosis		
Electrolyte abnormalities				
➤ **Hypo/hypernatraemia**				

Additional Systemic categories:

Drugs
- ➤ **Benzodiazepines**
- ➤ **Opiates**
- ➤ Anticonvulsants
- ➤ Antipsychotics
- ➤ Tricyclic antidepressants
- ➤ Anticholinergics
- ➤ Serotonin syndrome
- ➤ Neuroleptic malignant syndrome
- ➤ Miscellaneous

Toxins
- ➤ **Carbon monoxide**
- ➤ Ethylene glycol
- ➤ Methanol
- ➤ Solvent abuse
- ➤ Organophosphates
- ➤ Heavy metals
- ➤ Miscellaneous

Hypertensive disorders
- ➤ **Hypertensive encephalopathy**
- ➤ PRES
- ➤ Pre-eclampsia
- ➤ Eclampsia
- ➤ HELLP syndrome

Environmental
- ➤ Hypothermia

Table 6.1 Causes of coma or reduced level of consciousness – *continued*

Systemic	Local Infection	Vascular disease	Inflammation	Miscellaneous
➤ **Hypo/hypercalcaemia** ➤ Hypo/hypermagnesaemia ➤ Hypophosphataemia ➤ Hypokalaemia Inherited metabolic disorders ➤ Urea cycle disorders ➤ Disorders of amino acid metabolism ➤ Miscellaneous Nutritional deficiency ➤ **Wernicke–Korsakoff syndrome** ➤ **Vitamin B$_{12}$ deficiency** ➤ Pyridoxine deficiency ➤ Pellagra Alcohol-related diseases ➤ **Ethanol intoxication** ➤ **Delirium tremens** ➤ Marchiafava–Bignami disease	Focal CNS infection ➤ Intracranial abscess ➤ Bacterial cerebritis ➤ Cerebral sinus infection ➤ Subdural empyema ➤ Tuberculoma ➤ Intracranial fungal infection ➤ Toxoplasmosis ➤ Cysticercosis ➤ Hydatid disease ➤ Miscellaneous	➤ Susac's syndrome ➤ CADASIL ➤ Miscellaneous Posterior fossa arteriovenous malformation		

➤ alcohol intake
➤ foreign travel
➤ family history.

EXAMINATION
➤ Vital signs, including pulse, blood pressure, respiratory rate, temperature and oxygen saturation.
➤ Glasgow Coma Scale (GCS) score. This is a standardised method of measuring a patient's level of consciousness. It has three components, each of which is allocated a score as follows:

Motor response	
Obeys commands	6
Localises to pain	5
Withdraws from pain	4
Flexion to pain	3
Extension to pain	2
No response	1

Verbal response	
Normal speech	5
Confused speech	4
Inappropriate words	3
Incomprehensible sounds	2
No verbal response	1

Eye opening	
Open spontaneously	4
Open to voice	3
Open to pain	2
No eye opening	1

The GCS score is the total score, which can range from 3 to 15.
➤ Capillary blood glucose.
➤ General inspection, noting in particular any skin rash (meningococcal sepsis), jaundice (hepatic encephalopathy), cyanosis, cherry red skin (carbon monoxide poisoning), needle tracks (intravenous drug abuse), buccal or skin crease pigmentation (primary adrenal insufficiency), hypothyroid facies or evidence of head injury.
➤ Note the pattern of respiration. Slow and shallow breathing is associated with opiate or benzodiazepine poisoning, deep sighing breathing occurs with metabolic acidosis, particularly due to diabetic ketoacidosis, and Cheynes–Stokes (periodic) breathing occurs with brainstem lesions.
➤ The smell of the breath may give diagnostic clues. The smell of alcohol suggests intoxication, whereas that of ketones suggests diabetic ketoacidosis.
➤ Check for a flapping tremor of the outstretched hands with the wrists cocked back. This is usually caused by uraemia, hepatic encephalopathy or hypercarbia.
➤ Check for neck stiffness (which suggests meningitis), but do not manipulate the neck if there is any suspicion of cervical spine injury, or if the patient may have other cervical spine pathology such as atlanto-axial subluxation.
➤ Examine the pupils. Bilaterally constricted pupils occur with opiate poisoning and pontine lesions. Bilaterally dilated pupils occur with tricyclic antidepressant, anticholinergic or organophosphate poisoning, as well as with some brainstem lesions. Unilateral dilatation suggests transtentorial herniation due to raised intracranial pressure.
➤ Observe any spontaneous eye movements. Nystagmus may occur with cerebellar or brainstem lesions.
➤ Perform fundoscopy. Papilloedema is a sign of raised intracranial pressure, whereas subhyaloid haemorrhages may be seen in association with subarachnoid haemorrhage.
➤ Check the ears for haemotympanum, which is a sign of basal skull fracture.
➤ Examine limb tone and reflexes and check the plantar responses.

INVESTIGATIONS
The following core investigations are commonly required:
➤ Blood tests:
  – FBC and CRP. Raised WBC and CRP are features of infection.
  – U&Es and LFTs. Renal or hepatic failure may cause confusion or coma.
  – Calcium levels. Both hypo- and hypercalcaemia are possible causes of reduced level of consciousness.
  – INR. Abnormal clotting is a feature of fulminant hepatic failure.

- TFTs.
- Vitamin B_{12} levels.
- Serum osmolality is raised in hyperosmolar non-ketotic state and in poisoning by ethanol, methanol or ethylene glycol.
➤ Blood culture should be performed if sepsis is a possibility.
➤ ABG may reveal metabolic or respiratory acidosis.
➤ Urinalysis and urine MC&S may reveal urinary sepsis.
➤ Pregnancy test.
➤ ECG. Cardiac arrhythmias may cause shock and thus reduced cerebral perfusion.
➤ CXR. Aspiration is a common complication of reduced conscious level.
➤ CT of the head may reveal a variety of pathologies, including intracranial haemorrhage and space-occupying lesions.
➤ Lumbar puncture should be performed if meningitis or encephalitis is a possibility, but only after raised intracranial pressure has been ruled out by CT of the head and fundoscopy. Lumbar puncture in the presence of raised intracranial pressure may cause brainstem herniation through the foramen magnum, and death. Send CSF for:
  - glucose and protein
  - microscopy and culture
  - meningococcal and herpes simplex virus PCR
  - acid-fast bacilli (if tuberculous meningitis is suspected)
  - India ink staining (if cryptococcal meningitis is suspected)
  - cytology.

The following further investigations may be required:
➤ HIV test.
➤ Viral, syphilis or toxoplasma serology.
➤ Blood ammonia. This is raised with hepatic encephalopathy and urea cycle disorders.
➤ Blood and urine toxicology screen.
➤ Urinary porphyrins. These are raised with acute porphyria.
➤ Autoantibodies. These include ANA, ENA, anti-dsDNA (SLE), ANCA (Wegener's granulomatosis, Churg–Strauss syndrome), anti-TPO (Hashimoto's encephalopathy), anti-VGKC (non-paraneoplastic limbic encephalitis) and ANNA-1 (paraneoplastic limbic encephalitis).
➤ Short tetracosactide test. This may be diagnostic of adrenal insufficiency.
➤ Blood film. The intracellular parasites of malaria and African trypanosomiasis may be seen, while red cell fragments are characteristic of TTP.
➤ Serum viscosity. This is raised with hyperviscosity syndrome.
➤ Electroencephalogram. This is abnormal in status epilepticus.
➤ MRI of the brain. This is more sensitive than CT of the head for posterior fossa lesions and viral encephalitis. MR angiogram may visualise arterial dissection or occlusion, or evidence of cerebral vasculitis.

REFERENCE
1   Lora-Tamayo J, Palom X, Sarra J *et al*. Multiple myeloma and hyperammonemic encephalopathy: review of 27 cases. *Clin Lymph Myeloma*. 2008; 8(6): 363–9.

CHAPTER 7

Acute kidney injury

PATHOPHYSIOLOGY AND AETIOLOGY

The functions of the kidney include:
➤ excretion of waste products of metabolism
➤ regulation of extracellular volume, total body water content and electrolytes
➤ regulation of acid–base balance
➤ production of erythropoietin and 1,25-OH cholecalciferol.

Acute kidney injury (AKI) is diagnosed on the basis of an acute rise in serum creatinine concentration, a fall in glomerular filtration rate or a fall in urine output. AKI may be caused by a drop in renal perfusion (pre-renal AKI), obstruction to urine outflow at any point from the ureters to the urethral outlet (post-renal AKI), or intrinsic disease of the kidneys (renal AKI). Intrinsic renal disease may be further sub-divided into vascular disease, glomerular disease, acute interstitial nephritis and acute tubular necrosis.

Thus the mechanisms of acute kidney injury may be summarised as follows:
➤ pre-renal
➤ post-renal
➤ renal:
 – vascular disease
 – glomerular disease
 – acute interstitial nephritis
 – acute tubular necrosis.

The causes of acute kidney injury are listed in Table 7.1, with common causes highlighted in bold type.

EMERGENCY MANAGEMENT

Initial management focuses on the detection and treatment of life-threatening complications of acute kidney injury, and correction of easily reversible causes of renal dysfunction, such as hypovolaemia and urinary tract obstruction. Treatment priorities are as follows.
➤ Assess and treat disturbances of airway, breathing and circulation.
➤ Measure the serum potassium level urgently. Hyperkalaemia may cause asystole and cardiac arrest. Treat hyperkalaemia with IV calcium gluconate to protect the myocardium and an insulin/dextrose infusion to acutely lower the serum potassium level. Intractable hyperkalaemia is an indication for dialysis.
➤ Check for other life-threatening complications such as pulmonary oedema, uraemic pericarditis and uraemic encephalopathy. These are indications for urgent dialysis.
➤ Assess clinically for hypovolaemia, and provide fluid resuscitation if appropriate.
➤ Check for and treat sepsis.
➤ Check for urinary tract obstruction. Examine the abdomen for a distended bladder and arrange a renal tract USS. Relieve lower urinary tract obstruction with urethral or suprapubic catheterisation, and higher urinary tract obstruction with nephrostomy.
➤ Stop nephrotoxic drugs, including aminoglycoside antibiotics (consider alternative antimicrobials), ACE inhibitors, angiotensin II receptor blockers and NSAIDs.
➤ Investigate and treat the underlying cause.

HISTORY

➤ Nausea, vomiting, pruritus, malaise or lethargy are symptoms of uraemia.
➤ Fever, night sweats, weight loss, rash or arthralgia suggest systemic inflammation.
➤ Perform a full systemic enquiry, as multi-system disease may present with acute kidney injury.
➤ Ask about the quantity of urine being passed and its characteristics.
 – Macroscopic haematuria may be a sign of renal tract calculi or malignancy, as well as some glomerulonephritides.
 – Frothy urine occurs with proteinuria, a feature of glomerular disease.
 – Offensive urine suggests urinary tract infection.
➤ Dysuria suggests urinary tract infection or bladder calculi.
➤ Loin pain occurs with pyelonephritis, ureteric calculi and renal infarction.

Table 7.1 Causes of acute kidney injury

Pre-renal	Post-renal	Renal			
		Vascular disease	*Glomerular disease*	*Acute interstitial nephritis*	*Acute tubular necrosis*
Hypovolaemia ➤ Haemorrhage ➤ Diarrhoea ➤ Vomiting ➤ Bowel obstruction ➤ Ileus ➤ Pancreatitis ➤ Excessive diuresis ➤ Burns ➤ Heat illness ➤ Miscellaneous Generalised hypoperfusion ➤ Shock ➤ Sepsis ➤ Cardiac failure ➤ Hepatorenal syndrome Renal arterial disease ➤ Thromboembolism ➤ Stenosis ➤ Dissection ➤ Arteritis	Urethral ➤ Benign prostatic hypertrophy ➤ Prostate cancer ➤ Urethral stricture ➤ Urethral cancer ➤ Pinhole meatus ➤ Phimosis Vesical ➤ Bladder cancer ➤ Bladder calculi ➤ Neurogenic bladder Ureteric obstruction (luminal) ➤ Ureteric calculi ➤ Papillary necrosis ➤ Fungus ball Ureteric obstruction (mural) ➤ Pelviureteric cancer ➤ Ureteric stricture ➤ Surgical damage ➤ Pelviureteric neuromuscular dysfunction Ureteric obstruction (extrinsic) ➤ Retroperitoneal fibrosis ➤ Cervical cancer ➤ Rectal cancer ➤ Aortic aneurysm ➤ Retrocaval ureter	Microangiopathy ➤ Malignant hypertension ➤ Systemic sclerosis ➤ TTP/HUS ➤ Pre-eclampsia ➤ Eclampsia ➤ HELLP syndrome ➤ Antiphospholipid syndrome ➤ Cholesterol embolism Renal vein thrombosis	Primary glomerulopathies ➤ Goodpasture's disease ➤ IgA nephropathy ➤ Membranous nephropathy ➤ Mesangiocapillary glomerulonephritis Vasculitis ➤ Wegener's granulomatosis ➤ Churg–Strauss syndrome ➤ Microscopic polyangiitis ➤ Henoch–Schönlein purpura ➤ Cryoglobulinaemia ➤ Renal-limited vasculitis Connective tissue disease ➤ Systemic lupus erythematosus ➤ Rheumatoid arthritis ➤ Mixed connective tissue disease Infection ➤ Post-streptococcal glomerulonephritis ➤ Infective endocarditis ➤ Malaria ➤ Schistosomiasis ➤ HIV-associated nephropathy ➤ Miscellaneous	Drugs ➤ NSAIDs ➤ Antibiotics ➤ Diuretics ➤ Miscellaneous Infection ➤ Pyonephrosis ➤ Hantavirus ➤ Leptospirosis ➤ Legionella ➤ Tuberculosis ➤ Miscellaneous Inflammatory/autoimmune ➤ Systemic lupus erythematosus ➤ Sjögren's syndrome ➤ Sarcoidosis ➤ TINU syndrome ➤ Renal transplant rejection Malignant infiltration ➤ Leukaemia ➤ Lymphoma ➤ Miscellaneous	Ischaemic acute tubular necrosis Drugs ➤ Radiographic contrast media ➤ Aminoglycosides ➤ ACE inhibitors ➤ Angiotensin–receptor antagonists ➤ NSAIDs ➤ Lithium ➤ Miscellaneous Endogenous toxins ➤ Rhabdomyolysis ➤ Multiple myeloma ➤ POEMS syndrome ➤ Waldenström's macroglobulinaemia ➤ Plasma cell leukaemia ➤ Intravascular haemolysis ➤ Tumour lysis syndrome ➤ Hyperuricaemia ➤ Hypercalcaemia Exogenous toxins ➤ Toxic mushrooms ➤ Toxic plants ➤ Envenomation ➤ Ethylene glycol ➤ Heavy metals ➤ Organic solvents ➤ Chinese herbs

Pre-renal

Post-renal

- ⋏ Aberrant vessels
- ⋏ Adhesions
- ⋏ Diverticulitis
- ⋏ Crohn's disease
- ⋏ Pancreatitis
- ⋏ Pregnancy
- ⋏ Miscellaneous

Renal

Vascular disease

Glomerular disease

Miscellaneous
- ⋏ Amyloidosis
- ⋏ Monoclonal immunoglobulin deposition disease
- ⋏ Immunotactoid glomerulonephritis
- ⋏ Lipoprotein glomerulopathy

Acute interstitial nephritis

Acute tubular necrosis

- ⋏ Analgesic nephropathy
- ⋏ Heroin-associated nephropathy
- ⋏ Miscellaneous

Radiation nephropathy

➤ Urinary hesitancy, frequency or urgency, poor stream and terminal dribbling are features of prostatic enlargement.
➤ Recent sore throat may suggest post-streptococcal glomerulonephritis.
➤ Past medical history.
➤ Detailed drug history, including herbal and complementary remedies.
➤ Occupation, hobbies and foreign travel.
➤ Family history.

EXAMINATION
➤ Check the vital signs, including pulse, blood pressure, respiratory rate, temperature, oxygen saturations, urine output and GCS.
➤ General examination may reveal a skin rash, which suggests systemic infection or inflammation. Also check for a uraemic flap.
➤ Assess the fluid status. Signs of hypovolaemia include tachycardia, tachypnoea, hypotension, postural hypotension, prolonged capillary refill time, cool peripheries, weak thready pulse, dry mucous membranes and reduced skin turgor. Signs of fluid overload include raised JVP, peripheral or sacral oedema, ascites and fine crackles at the lung bases.
➤ Auscultate the heart, listening specifically for a pericardial rub, which suggests uraemic pericarditis.
➤ Abdominal examination may reveal a palpable bladder (due to bladder outflow obstruction) or enlarged kidneys (due to polycystic kidney disease or hydronephrosis).
➤ Perform a full neurological examination. Neurological abnormalities in association with renal failure may be due to thrombotic thrombocytopaenic purpura.

INVESTIGATIONS
The following core investigations are commonly required:
➤ Urine dip:
  – Proteinuria occurs with glomerular disease.
  – Proteinuria with haematuria suggests glomerulonephritis.
  – Isolated haematuria may be due to renal tract malignancy or calculi.
  – Nitrites and leucocytes are features of urinary tract infection.
➤ Urine MC&S:
  – Red cell casts are diagnostic of glomerulonephritis.
  – White cells or micro-organisms are seen with urinary tract infection.
  – Culture and sensitivities may reveal infection.
➤ Blood tests:
  – U&Es.
  – FBC. Anaemia may be a consequence of chronic renal impairment, or systemic inflammation or infection. A raised WBC suggests infection.
  – CRP. This is raised with infection.
  – LFTs. Hepatic failure may lead to the hepatorenal syndrome.
  – Phosphate. Hyperphosphataemia is a common feature of acute kidney injury.
  – Calcium. Chronic renal failure is often associated with hypocalcaemia due to vitamin D deficiency. Hypercalcaemia with renal failure suggests multiple myeloma.
  – Bicarbonate. This allows assessment of the acid–base status.
  – Albumin. Levels are low in nephrotic syndrome.
  – CK. Levels are raised with rhabdomyolysis.
  – Urate. Levels are raised with gouty nephropathy.
➤ CXR. This may reveal airspace shadowing due to pulmonary oedema, alveolar haemorrhage (secondary to vasculitis) or pneumonia.
➤ ECG. Tall tented T-waves, widened QRS complexes and a prolonged PR interval are signs of severe hyperkalaemia that requires urgent treatment.
➤ USS of the renal tract may show hydronephrosis, which suggests urinary tract obstruction. Doppler may be used to detect renal artery or vein occlusion.

The following further investigations may be required:
➤ PSA. This may be raised with benign prostatic hypertrophy or prostate cancer.
➤ Connective tissue and vasculitis screen:
  – ANA, ENA and RhF
  – anti-dsDNA (systemic lupus erythematosus)
  – ANCA (Wegener's granulomatosis, Churg–Strauss syndrome)
  – anti-GBM antibody (Goodpasture's disease)
  – anti-cardiolipin antibodies, lupus anticoagulant and anti-b2 glycoprotein I (antiphospholipid syndrome)
  – complement components C3 and C4 (which are low in systemic lupus erythematosus)
  – cryoglobulins.

➤ Serum electrophoresis, serum free light chains and urinary Bence Jones proteins are required to diagnose plasma cell dyscrasias such as multiple myeloma.
➤ Serology:
   – HIV
   – hepatitis B and C (associated with polyarteritis nodosa and cryoglobulinaemia, respectively)
   – anti-streptolysin O titre (positive in post-streptococcal glomerulonephritis).
➤ Blood film may show red cell fragments, which suggests a microangiopathic haemolytic anaemia such as thrombotic thrombocytopaenic purpura.
➤ Urinary sodium may be useful to help to distinguish between pre-renal acute kidney injury (usually < 20 mmol/l) and acute tubular necrosis (usually > 40 mmol/l).[1]
➤ Imaging:
   – CT of the kidneys, ureters and bladder allows urinary tract calculi and mass lesions to be visualised
   – renal MR angiogram is the investigation of choice for detecting renal artery stenosis.
➤ Renal biopsy may be necessary to diagnose intrinsic renal disease.

REFERENCE

1   Miller TR, Anderson RJ, Linas SL. Urinary diagnostic indices in acute renal failure. *Ann Intern Med.* 1978; **89**: 47–50.

CHAPTER 8

Pleuritic chest pain

PATHOPHYSIOLOGY AND AETIOLOGY

Pain in general may be divided into three categories, namely somatic, visceral and neuropathic. Somatic pain arises from superficial structures such as the skin, ribs and intercostal muscles, as well as the parietal pleura and pericardium. It is transmitted by fast-conducting A-delta fibres, and is typically sharp in character and well localised. Visceral pain arises from the internal organs and is transmitted by slow-conducting C fibres. It is typically dull or aching in character and poorly localised. Neuropathic pain is caused by injury to the peripheral nerves, spinal cord or brain. It may have a number of characteristics, ranging from lancinating to burning in nature.

Pleuritic chest pain refers to pain arising from pleural irritation. It is characterically sharp in nature, well localised and exacerbated by inspiration, and is thus a form of somatic pain, mediated by fast-conducting A-delta fibres. Since pain with very similar characteristics may result from pathology affecting the chest wall or pericardium, these conditions are best discussed together. For the purposes of this chapter, the term 'pleuritic chest pain' will be used to refer to any chest pain that is sharp, well localised and exacerbated by inspiration, regardless of its origin.

The causes of pleuritic chest pain may be classified into pleural and non-pleural categories, as shown in Table 8.1.

EMERGENCY MANAGEMENT

➤ Potentially life-threatening causes of pleuritic chest pain include pulmonary embolism (PE), tension pneumothorax, pneumonia and empyema.
➤ If pulmonary embolism is suspected clinically, anticoagulation with low-molecular-weight heparin should be initiated immediately, unless contraindicated, pending further investigation. Massive PE causing haemodynamic compromise should be treated with thrombolysis unless there is a contraindication.[1]
➤ Tension pneumothorax is an immediately life-threatening cause of pleuritic chest pain. A patient with tension pneumothorax will be extremely tachypnoeic and tachycardic, and deteriorating rapidly. There may be cyanosis or hypotension. On examination of the chest there will be reduced expansion, absent breath sounds and hyper-resonance to percussion on the ipsilateral side, with tracheal deviation away from the side of the pneumothorax. The jugular venous pressure may be raised. A tension pneumothorax should be diagnosed clinically, and then immediately decompressed by inserting a large-bore cannula into the ipsilateral pleural cavity at the second intercostal space in the mid-clavicular line. A rush of air will be heard. An intercostal drain should then be inserted.
➤ Bacterial pneumonia and empyema should be treated with timely antibiotic therapy. In cases of pleural infection, intercostal tube insertion and pleural fluid drainage are indicated if the fluid has a pH of less than 7.2 or is purulent.[2]

HISTORY

➤ Record the characteristics of the pain.
  – Site and radiation. Pleuritic pain may occur anywhere on the chest wall, but is by definition well localised. The pain of pericarditis is typically retrosternal, with possible radiation to the back.
  – Character and severity. Pleuritic chest pain is by definition sharp in character, and may range from mild to extremely severe.

Table 8.1 Causes of pleuritic chest pain

Pleural
Pneumothorax

Infection
➤ Pneumonia
➤ Empyema
➤ Lung abscess
➤ Tuberculosis
➤ Miscellaneous

Pulmonary infarction
➤ Pulmonary embolism
➤ Sickle-cell chest crisis
➤ Decompression sickness

Malignancy
➤ Lung cancer
➤ Malignant mesothelioma
➤ Metastatic malignancy
➤ Lymphoma
➤ Leukaemia
➤ Miscellaneous

Connective tissue disease
➤ Systemic lupus erythematosus
➤ Rheumatoid arthritis
➤ Mixed connective tissue disease
➤ Sjögren's syndrome
➤ Adult Still's disease

Vasculitis
➤ Churg–Strauss syndrome
➤ Wegener's granulomatosis
➤ Polyarteritis nodosa
➤ Giant-cell arteritis

Extrinsic insults
➤ Benign asbestos pleural effusion
➤ Drug-induced pleuritis
➤ Serum sickness
➤ Radiation pleuritis
➤ Electrical injury

Subdiaphragmatic pathology
➤ Acute pancreatitis
➤ Acute cholecystitis
➤ Subphrenic abscess
➤ Hepatic abscess
➤ Fitz–Hugh–Curtis syndrome
➤ Peritonitis

Miscellaneous
➤ Oesophageal rupture
➤ Mediastinitis
➤ Haemothorax
➤ Chylothorax
➤ Urinothorax
➤ Biliothorax
➤ Meig's syndrome
➤ Dressler's syndrome
➤ Familial Mediterranean fever
➤ Whipple's disease
➤ Endometriosis
➤ Yellow nail syndrome
➤ Pulmonary alveolar proteinosis
➤ Eosinophilic pneumonia
➤ Lymphomatoid granulomatosis
➤ Sarcoidosis
➤ Berylliosis
➤ Uraemia
➤ OHSS

Extra-pleural
Acute pericarditis
➤ Malignant
➤ Viral
➤ Bacterial
➤ Tuberculous
➤ Fungal
➤ Inflammatory
➤ Miscellaneous

Asthma

Chest wall trauma
➤ Muscle tear
➤ Rib fracture

Chest wall inflammation
➤ Costochondritis
➤ Systemic lupus erythematosus
➤ Rheumatoid arthritis
➤ Ankylosing spondylitis
➤ Psoriatic arthritis
➤ Reactive arthritis
➤ Enteropathic arthritis
➤ SAPHO syndrome
➤ Relapsing polychondritis
➤ Sickle-cell bone crisis

Musculoskeletal infection
➤ Osteomyelitis
➤ Bornholm disease

Malignant bone infiltration
➤ Multiple myeloma
➤ Bone metastases
➤ Primary bone malignancy
➤ Miscellaneous

- Time and mode of onset. Instantaneous onset associated with trauma or heavy lifting suggests a musculoskeletal cause. Most causes of pleural inflammation develop over a period of hours to days.
- Exacerbating factors. Pleuritic pain is by definition exacerbated by inspiration. Pain that is made worse by chest wall movement to a greater extent than by breathing is likely to be musculoskeletal in origin, but serious pathology such as pulmonary embolism cannot be ruled out solely on this basis. Pericardial pain is classically worse on lying flat, and relieved by sitting forward.
➤ Associated symptoms:
  - Dyspnoea or cough suggests a primary pleural or pulmonary pathology (e.g. pneumothorax, pulmonary embolism or pneumonia).
  - Leg pain or swelling suggests deep vein thrombosis with subsequent pulmonary embolism.
➤ Risk factors for PE should be inquired about. Major risk factors include recent orthopaedic or other major surgery, lower limb fractures, varicose veins, immobility, previous venous thromboembolism, advanced or abdomino-pelvic malignancy, and late pregnancy or the puerperium. Minor risk factors include use of the combined oral contraceptive pill, and chronic medical conditions such as congestive cardiac failure and chronic obstructive pulmonary disease.[1]

EXAMINATION
➤ Record the vital signs, including pulse, blood pressure, respiratory rate, temperature and oxygen saturation.
➤ Assess the jugular venous pressure (JVP). Raised JVP occurs with haemodynamically significant pericardial effusions, massive pulmonary embolism and tension pneumothorax.
➤ Check for pulsus paradoxus (a fall in systolic blood pressure of more than 10 mmHg on inspiration). This occurs with cardiac tamponade, a possible consequence of a large pericardial effusion.

➤ Carefully palpate the chest wall for local tenderness, in particular noting whether such palpation reproduces the patient's pain. Severe tenderness to light palpation suggests a musculoskeletal cause. However, one pitfall is that pleural irritation (e.g. due to a pulmonary embolism) may also cause chest wall tenderness due to movement of the underlying pleura.

➤ Check the tracheal position. It will be deviated away from the side of a tension pneumothorax or massive pleural effusion.

➤ Percuss and auscultate the chest. Bronchial breathing or coarse crackles suggests pneumonia. Dullness to percussion, reduced breath sounds and reduced vocal resonance occur with pleural effusion. Hyper-resonance to percussion, reduced breath sounds and reduced vocal resonance are signs of pneumothorax.

➤ Palpate and auscultate the precordium. Massive pulmonary embolism may cause a loud or even palpable pulmonary second heart sound. A pericardial rub may be present with acute pericarditis.

➤ Inspect the legs for swelling or tenderness that may indicate deep vein thrombosis and subsequent pulmonary embolism.

INVESTIGATIONS
The following core investigations are commonly required:

➤ CXR. This may reveal pneumonia, pleural effusion, pneumothorax or rib fracture.

➤ ECG. Pulmonary embolism most commonly causes sinus tachycardia, but signs of right heart strain such as right bundle branch block or right axis deviation may be seen. Low voltage complexes or widespread saddle-shaped ST elevation with PR depression suggests a pericardial effusion.

➤ ABG. This is not required in all cases, but the presence of a raised alveolar–arterial oxygen gradient suggests significant pulmonary pathology, such as pulmonary embolism.

➤ D-dimer. This blood test should be performed if pulmonary embolism is a reasonable possibility. It is sensitive for PE, but rather non-specific. Therefore a negative test (using a sensitive D-dimer assay) in a patient at low or medium risk of PE reliably rules out the diagnosis.[1] However, a patient at high risk must be investigated further with a CT pulmonary angiogram (CTPA) or ventilation/perfusion (V/Q) scan, regardless of the D-dimer result.

There are a number of scoring systems available to aid the clinician in classifying patients into low-, intermediate- or high-risk categories for PE. These include the Geneva and Wells scores. A simpler scheme, recommended by the British Thoracic Society, is based on only two questions:

1   Is there a major risk factor for pulmonary embolism?
2   Is there an absence of another reasonable clinical explanation for the symptoms?

Patients score a point for each positive answer, and are classified into low-, intermediate- or high-risk categories according to whether they score 0, 1 or 2 points, respectively.[1]
The following further investigations may be required:

➤ CTPA or V/Q scan. If the patient has a high clinical probability of pulmonary embolism, or if the D-dimer is positive, a CTPA or V/Q scan should be performed to confirm or exclude the diagnosis. A CTPA has the advantage of being able to diagnose alternative causes of the symptoms, such as pneumonia, but the radiation dose to the patient is higher. CTPA is the investigation of choice if there is underlying pulmonary disease or the CXR is abnormal, as V/Q scanning is unlikely to be diagnostic in this instance. The majority of clinicians feel that CTPA is preferable to V/Q scanning in pregnancy, as the radiation dose to the fetus is reduced. However, there is theoretical concern that irradiation of the breast during pregnancy may increase the risk of breast cancer later in life.[3]

➤ Leg venous Doppler. Pregnant women with suspected pulmonary embolism should undergo a bilateral leg Doppler scan before undergoing a CTPA or V/Q scan, as a positive diagnosis of deep vein thrombosis will necessitate anticoagulation in any case, and thus obviate the need to expose the mother and fetus to ionising radiation.

➤ Thoracocentesis is required for the diagnosis of a pleural effusion. The pleural fluid should be analysed for the following:
  – pH.
  – Protein and LDH. Pleural effusions are classified as exudates or transudates. Exudates are protein-rich, with a high LDH, and are caused by pleural infection, inflammation or neoplasia. Transudates are low in protein, with a low LDH, and are caused by haemodynamic factors such as congestive cardiac failure.
  – MC&S and Ziehl–Neelsen stain are required to diagnose bacterial or mycobacterial infection.
  – Cytology may be diagnostic of pleural malignancy.

➤ Echocardiogram. Massive pulmonary embolism may cause right heart strain with raised pulmonary artery pressure. Pericardial effusion can also be seen if present.

➤ Autoantibody screen (ANA, ENA, RhF and ANCA). This should be requested if connective tissue disease or vasculitis is suspected as a cause of pleural or pericardial inflammation.

➤ Viral serology. This may be diagnostic of viral pericarditis or Bornholm disease.

REFERENCES

1   British Thoracic Society Standards of Care Committee Pulmonary Embolism Guideline Development Group. British Thoracic Society guidelines for the management of suspected acute pulmonary embolism. *Thorax.* 2003; **58**: 470–84.
2   Davies CWH, Gleeson FV, Davies RJO. BTS guidelines for the management of pleural infection. *Thorax.* 2003; **58 (Suppl. II):** ii18–28.
3   Matthews S. Imaging pulmonary embolism in pregnancy: what is the most appropriate imaging protocol? *Br J Radiol.* 2006; **79**: 441–4.

CHAPTER 9

Non-pleuritic chest pain

PATHOPHYSIOLOGY AND AETIOLOGY

Pleuritic chest pain (*see* Chapter 8) is characterised by being well localised, sharp in nature and exacerbated by inspiration. Chest pain that does not have these characteristics is described as non-pleuritic.

Non-pleuritic chest pain may be caused by a number of different mechanisms, including the following:

➤ myocardial ischaemia
➤ pericardial irritation
➤ aortic injury or inflammation
➤ upper respiratory tract irritation
➤ upper gastrointestinal tract irritation
➤ oesophageal spasm
➤ diaphragmatic irritation
➤ chest wall injury or inflammation
➤ neuropathic pain
➤ functional causes.

The causes of non-pleuritic chest pain are listed in Table 9.1, with common causes highlighted in bold type.

EMERGENCY MANAGEMENT

➤ The main focus of investigation should be on diagnosing or excluding an acute coronary syndrome. Other serious, but less common, causes of acute chest pain include aortic dissection and oesophageal rupture.
➤ ST elevation myocardial infarction (STEMI) is caused by complete occlusion of a main coronary artery. Initial management is as follows.[1]
  – Ensure that the airway, breathing and circulation are secure.
  – Correct hypoxia with high-flow oxygen if necessary.
  – Give aspirin 300 mg and clopidogrel 300 mg orally.
  – Render the patient pain-free if possible with sublingual GTN and IV morphine. Consider a GTN infusion if the patient is still not pain-free.
  – Administer a β-blocker if there are no contraindications such as heart failure, pulse < 60 beats per minute, systolic blood pressure < 100 mmHg, severe airways disease or conduction defects.
  – Ensure tight glycaemic control using an insulin infusion in diabetic or hyperglycaemic patients. This has been shown to reduce mortality.[2]
  – PCI is the reperfusion therapy of choice if it is available. Otherwise, thrombolysis should be given if it is not contraindicated. Reperfusion therapy should be provided as quickly as possible in order to avoid extensive myocardial necrosis. Thrombolysis should ideally be performed within 30 minutes of presentation, and PCI within 90 minutes of presentation.
➤ Non-ST elevation myocardial infarction (NSTEMI) and unstable angina are caused by an unstable ruptured coronary plaque. Initial management is as follows.[1]
  – Ensure that the airway, breathing and circulation are secure.
  – Give oxygen, aspirin, clopidogrel, GTN and morphine as with STEMI.
  – Give subcutaneous low-molecular-weight heparin.
  – Administer a β-blocker if there are no contraindications.
  – Ensure tight glycaemic control in diabetic or hyperglycaemic patients.
  – Proceed to early coronary angiography.
➤ Thoracic aortic dissection is categorised as type A, in which the dissection involves the ascending aorta, or type B, in which it does not. Type A dissection requires surgical treatment, whereas type B dissection is treated conservatively with tight blood pressure control and analgesia.
➤ Oesophageal rupture (referred to as Boerhaave's syndrome when spontaneous) requires vigorous fluid resuscitation, broad-spectrum antibiotics and urgent surgical intervention.

HISTORY

➤ A detailed description of the pain should be obtained, incorporating the following features. The characteristics of the different categories of chest pain are shown in Table 9.2, and can be summarised as follows:

- site and radiation
- character and severity
- time and mode of onset
- course and pattern
- previous episodes
- exacerbating factors
- relieving factors.

Table 9.1 Causes of non-pleuritic chest pain

Cardiovascular and respiratory		Abdominal	Musculoskeletal and neurological
Myocardial ischaemia	*Miscellaneous*	Oesophageal	Trauma
Angina pectoris	Acute pericarditis	➤ GORD	➤ Muscle tear
	➤ Malignant	➤ Oesophagitis	➤ Rib fracture
Acute coronary syndromes	➤ Viral	➤ Dysmotility	
➤ Unstable angina	➤ Bacterial	➤ Carcinoma	Inflammation
➤ NSTEMI	➤ Tuberculous	➤ Stenosis	➤ Costochondritis
➤ STEMI	➤ Fungal	➤ Rupture	➤ Systemic lupus
	➤ Inflammatory		erythematosus
Reduced oxygen delivery	➤ Miscellaneous	Gastroduodenal	➤ Rheumatoid arthritis
➤ Cardiac arrhythmia		➤ Gastritis	➤ Ankylosing spondylitis
➤ Hypoxia	Aortic pathology	➤ Peptic ulcer disease	➤ Psoriatic arthritis
➤ Shock	➤ Thoracic aortic		➤ Reactive arthritis
➤ Anaemia	dissection	Hepatobiliary/pancreatic	➤ Enteropathic arthritis
➤ Polycythaemia	➤ Aortic intramural	➤ Pancreatitis	➤ SAPHO syndrome
➤ Carbon monoxide	haematoma	➤ Acute cholecystitis	➤ Relapsing polychondritis
poisoning	➤ Penetrating aortic ulcer	➤ Acute cholangitis	➤ Sickle-cell crisis
➤ Cyanide poisoning	➤ Thoracic aortic aneurysm	➤ Biliary colic	
➤ Methaemoglobinaemia	➤ Aortitis	➤ Hepatitis	Infection
		➤ Hepatic abscess	➤ Osteomyelitis
Increased cardiac work	Respiratory	➤ Fitz–Hugh–Curtis	➤ Bornholm disease
➤ Aortic stenosis	➤ Asthma	syndrome	
➤ Aortic regurgitation	➤ Tracheobronchitis		Neoplasia
➤ Malignant hypertension	➤ Toxin inhalation	Miscellaneous	➤ Multiple myeloma
➤ Pulmonary hypertension		➤ Subphrenic abscess	➤ Bone metastases
➤ Hyperthyroidism		➤ Peritonitis	➤ Primary bone malignancy
➤ Phaeochromocytoma			➤ Mediastinal mass
➤ Beriberi			➤ Lung cancer
			➤ Miscellaneous
Myocardial disease			
➤ Hypertrophic			Breast pathology
cardiomyopathy			➤ Infection
➤ Dilated cardiomyopathy			➤ Trauma
➤ Peripartum			➤ Thrombophlebitis
cardiomyopathy			➤ Tumour
➤ Stress-induced			➤ Miscellaneous
cardiomyopathy			
➤ Myocarditis			Neuropathic pain
			➤ Shingles
Coronary artery damage			➤ Post-herpetic neuralgia
➤ Coronary artery			➤ Spinal radiculopathy
dissection			➤ Brachial plexus injury
➤ Kawasaki disease			➤ Transverse myelitis
➤ Takayasu arteritis			
			Functional
Coronary artery spasm			➤ Hyperventilation
➤ Prinzmetal angina			➤ Fibromyalgia
➤ Sumatriptan			➤ Miscellaneous
➤ Nicotine			
➤ Amphetamines			
➤ MDMA			
➤ Cocaine			

Table 9.2 Characteristics of chest pain by aetiology

	Site and radiation	Character	Onset	Associated symptoms	Exacerbating factors	Relieving factors
Myocardial ischaemia	Anterior chest with radiation to the arms, jaws or back	Diffuse, crushing or aching	Variable	Sweating, pallor, malaise, anxiety, shortness of breath, nausea, vomiting	Exertion	Rest, nitrates
Pericardial irritation	Anterior chest with radiation to the back	Sharp, stabbing or aching	Variable		Lying supine	Leaning forwards
Aortic dissection	Upper back or anterior chest radiating to the back	Tearing or ripping; severe	Usually sudden	Focal sensory or motor deficits possible		
Pleural irritation	Variable	Sharp, stabbing	Variable	Shortness of breath, cough	Inspiration	
Upper respiratory tract irritation	Sub-sternal	Raw, burning	Hours to days	Cough	Coughing	
Upper gastrointestinal tract irritation	Anterior chest	Burning	Variable	Dyspepsia, abdominal pain, nausea or vomiting	Hot or spicy food, bending forward, lying flat	Milk, antacids
Oesophageal spasm	Anterior chest with radiation to the arms, jaws or back	Diffuse, crushing or aching	Seconds to minutes		Eating or drinking	GTN spray may relieve symptoms
Chest wall injury or inflammation	Variable	Well localised; sharp, stabbing or aching	May be associated injury or trauma		Movement, local pressure, inspiration	
Neuropathic	Back, radiating round to the anterior chest. Usually unilateral	Variable	Variable	Focal sensory or motor deficits	Movement may exacerbate	
Functional	Variable	Variable	Variable	Anxiety, palpitations, paraesthesiae		

➤ Associated symptoms:
  – Palpitation occurs with cardiac arrhythmias.
  – Dyspnoea may occur with myocardial ischaemia.
  – Cough suggests upper respiratory tract irritation.
  – Nausea or vomiting may occur with myocardial ischaemia or gastrointestinal pathology.
    Sweating is a common feature of myocardial ischaemia.
➤ Inquire about use of illicit drugs, particularly cocaine.
➤ Enquire about risk factors for coronary heart disease. These include hypertension, dyslipidaemia, diabetes mellitus, smoking, and a family history of coronary heart disease.

EXAMINATION
➤ Palpate the pulse, noting the rate, rhythm, character and volume. Radio-radial or radio-femoral delay may occur with aortic dissection.
➤ Check the blood pressure in both arms. A difference in the systolic blood pressure of more than 20 mmHg is a sign of possible aortic dissection.
➤ Assess the jugular venous pressure (JVP). Raised JVP may occur with a haemodynamically significant pericardial effusion or with myocardial infarction complicated by cardiac failure.
➤ Inspect and palpate the chest wall carefully for local tenderness and swelling. Tenderness and/or swelling over the costochondral joints suggest costochondritis, particularly if palpation reproduces the patient's pain. Tender spots in other areas of the chest may be associated with rib fractures, muscle tears or chest wall trauma. Check for the rash of shingles.

➤ Auscultate the heart. In particular, check for the ejection systolic murmur of aortic stenosis or hypertrophic cardiomyopathy, and the early diastolic murmur of aortic regurgitation, which may occur with aortic dissection.

➤ Palpate the abdomen. A number of pathologies, such as acute cholecystitis or acute pancreatitis, may cause abdominal pain that radiates into the chest. Abdominal tenderness or peritonism suggests intra-abdominal pathology.

INVESTIGATIONS
The following core investigations are commonly required:

➤ ECG. Signs of cardiac ischaemia include ST segment elevation or depression, and T-wave inversion. New-onset left bundle branch block is equivalent to ST elevation, and should be treated as such. Widespread saddle-shaped ST segment elevation, PR segment depression and small voltage complexes occur with acute pericarditis and pericardial effusions.

➤ CXR may reveal rib fractures, or a widened mediastinum associated with aortic dissection.

➤ Blood tests:
  – FBC. Severe anaemia may cause myocardial ischaemia.
  – LFTs. Hepatitis may cause abdominal pain that radiates to the chest.
  – CRP is a marker of infection or inflammation.
  – Amylase activity should be measured if pancreatitis is suspected.
  – Troponin levels are measured 12 hours after the time of maximal pain severity. Troponin is specific for myocardial damage, although this may not necessarily be due to a thrombotic coronary event. Myocardial damage and thus raised blood troponin levels may also be caused by congestive cardiac failure, pulmonary embolism, sepsis and a variety of other pathologies.[3] Troponin levels may also be raised in acute or chronic renal failure.

The following further investigations may be required:

➤ Echocardiogram. Impaired ventricular function may occur with myocardial ischaemia or myocarditis. Valvular lesions and pericardial effusions may also be detected.

➤ Exercise ECG. This is used to investigate patients in whom the history suggests cardiac ischaemia but the troponin levels and ECG are both normal. Chest pain and/or ischaemic ECG changes on exercise suggest coronary artery disease.

➤ Myocardial perfusion scan allows areas of reversible cardiac ischaemia to be visualised.

➤ Coronary angiography is used as both a therapeutic and diagnostic tool. In the acute setting, it is the most effective therapy for reperfusing the heart following an STEMI. Coronary angiography should be performed early after NSTEMI to detect and treat coronary artery stenotic lesions.

➤ CT of the chest is used to diagnose aortic dissection, and may also show bone infiltration or intrathoracic neoplasia.

➤ OGD may be required to diagnose oesophageal or gastric pathology.

➤ CT or USS of the abdomen should be performed if subdiaphragmatic pathology such as acute cholecystitis or pancreatitis is suspected.

➤ Viral serology may assist in the diagnosis of viral pericarditis, viral myocarditis or Bornholm disease.

REFERENCES
1 Scottish Intercollegiate Guidelines Network. *Acute Coronary Syndromes: SIGN Guideline 93*. Edinburgh: Scottish Intercollegiate Guidelines Network; 2007.

2 Malmberg K, Ryden L, Hamsten A *et al*. Randomized trial of insulin-glucose infusion followed by subcutaneous insulin treatment in diabetic patients with acute myocardial infarction (DIGAMI study): effects on mortality at 1 year. *J Am Coll Cardiol*. 1995; **26**: 57–65.

3 Jeremias A, Gibson CM. Narrative review: alternative causes for elevated cardiac troponin levels when acute coronary syndromes are excluded. *Ann Intern Med*. 2005; **142**: 786–91.

CHAPTER 10

Palpitation

PATHOPHYSIOLOGY AND AETIOLOGY

Palpitation may be defined as an abnormal awareness of one's own heartbeat. The diagnosis is considerably easier if the symptoms are present at the time of the patient's clinical assessment. In this instance, an ECG may reveal a cardiac arrhythmia, thus allowing the cause of the symptoms to be determined immediately. However, on many occasions the symptoms are episodic and have resolved by the time the patient seeks medical attention. Palpitation may result from two primary mechanisms:

➤ abnormal pulse rate or rhythm
➤ abnormally forceful cardiac contraction.

An abnormal pulse rate or rhythm may represent sinus tachycardia of any cause, or a cardiac arrhythmia. An abnormally forceful cardiac contraction occurs as a result of sympathetic system overactivity, which has a variety of causes, including hypoglycaemia and hyperthyroidism.

The causes of palpitation are summarised in Table 10.1, with common causes highlighted in bold type.

EMERGENCY TREATMENT

➤ Measure the pulse rate and blood pressure, and check for signs of cardiovascular compromise. These include reduced level of consciousness, chest pain that suggests cardiac ischaemia, and clinical features of congestive cardiac failure.
➤ Tachyarrhythmia causing severe hypotension (systolic blood pressure < 90 mmHg) or cardiovascular compromise should be treated with urgent electrical cardioversion. If the patient is still conscious, anaesthetic support will be required to provide the necessary level of sedation to deliver the DC shock. The recommended algorithm for the management of tachyarrhythmias, published by the Resuscitation Council (UK),[1] is shown in Figure 10.1.

Table 10.1 Causes of palpitation

Abnormal pulse rate or rhythm	Abnormally forceful cardiac contraction
Tachyarrhythmia	Anaemia
➤ Atrial fibrillation	
➤ Atrial flutter	Endocrine/metabolic
➤ Atrial tachycardia	➤ Hyperthyroidism
➤ Junctional tachycardia	➤ Hypoglycaemia
➤ Ventricular tachycardia	➤ Phaeochromocytoma
	➤ Carcinoid syndrome
Bradyarrhythmia	➤ Mastocytosis
➤ Second-degree heart block	➤ Beriberi
➤ Complete heart block	
	Drugs and toxins
Extrasystole	➤ Theophyllines
➤ Atrial	➤ Sympathomimetics
➤ Ventricular	➤ Caffeine
	➤ Nicotine
Miscellaneous	➤ Cocaine
➤ Postural orthostatic tachycardia syndrome	➤ Amphetamines
➤ Sinus tachycardia	➤ MDMA
	➤ Carbon monoxide poisoning
	➤ Scombrotoxic fish poisoning
	Psychological
	➤ Anxiety
	➤ Panic attack
	Structural cardiovascular abnormalities
	➤ Aortic regurgitation
	➤ Arteriovenous fistula

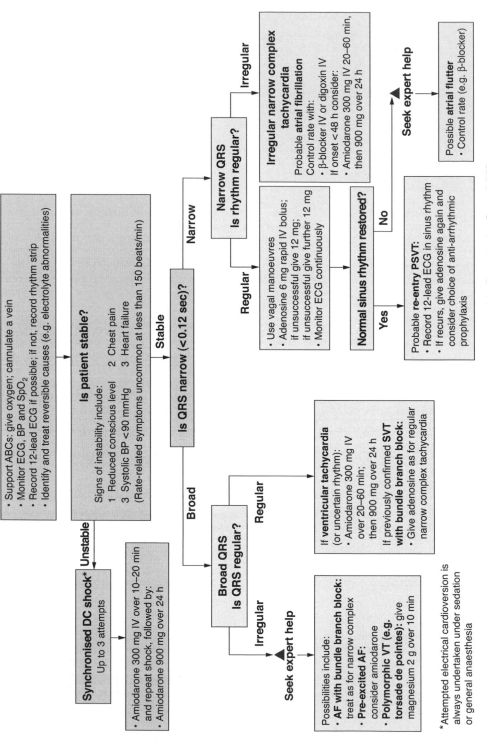

Figure 10.1 Algorithm for the management of tachycardia. Reproduced with kind permission of the Resuscitation Council (UK).

Support ABCs: give oxygen; cannulate a vein
- Monitor ECG, BP and SpO₂
- Record 12-lead ECG if possible; if not, record rhythm strip
- Identify and treat reversible causes (e.g. electrolyte abnormalities)

Is patient stable?

Signs of instability include:
1 Reduced conscious level   2 Chest pain
3 Systolic BP <90 mmHg   3 Heart failure
(Rate-related symptoms uncommon at less than 150 beats/min)

Unstable

Synchronised DC shock*
Up to 3 attempts

- Amiodarone 300 mg IV over 10–20 min and repeat shock, followed by:
- Amiodarone 900 mg over 24 h

Stable

Is QRS narrow (<0.12 sec)?

Broad

Broad QRS
Is QRS regular?

Regular

If **ventricular tachycardia** (or uncertain rhythm):
- Amiodarone 300 mg IV over 20–60 min; then 900 mg over 24 h
If previously confirmed **SVT with bundle branch block:**
- Give adenosine as for regular narrow complex tachycardia

Irregular

Seek expert help

Possibilities include:
- **AF with bundle branch block:** treat as for narrow complex
- **Pre-excited AF:** consider amiodarone
- **Polymorphic VT (e.g. torsade de pointes):** give magnesium 2 g over 10 min

Narrow

Narrow QRS
Is rhythm regular?

Regular

- Use vagal manoeuvres
- Adenosine 6 mg rapid IV bolus; if unsuccessful give 12 mg; if unsuccessful give further 12 mg
- Monitor ECG continuously

Normal sinus rhythm restored?

Yes

Probable **re-entry PSVT:**
- Record 12-lead ECG in sinus rhythm
- If recurs, give adenosine again and consider choice of anti-arrhythmic prophylaxis

No

Seek expert help

Irregular

Irregular narrow complex tachycardia

Probable **atrial fibrillation**
Control rate with:
- β-blocker IV or digoxin IV
If onset <48 h consider:
- Amiodarone 300 mg IV 20–60 min, then 900 mg over 24 h

Seek expert help

Possible **atrial flutter**
- Control rate (e.g. β-blocker)

*Attempted electrical cardioversion is always undertaken under sedation or general anaesthesia

➤ Bradyarrhythmia that is causing severe hypotension (systolic blood pressure < 90 mmHg), pulse rate of < 40 beats per minute or cardiovascular compromise should be treated initially with 500 micrograms of IV atropine, which may be repeated up to a total of 3 mg. If this is unsuccessful, transcutaneous or transvenous temporary pacing should be initiated. The recommended algorithm for the management of bradyarrhythmias, published by the Resuscitation Council (UK),[1] is shown in Figure 10.2.

HISTORY
➤ The following features may provide diagnostic clues.
  - Time and mode of onset of symptoms. Sinus tachycardia develops gradually, whereas cardiac arrhythmias usually begin suddenly.
  - Frequency of symptoms.
  - Duration of symptoms.
  - Character of palpitations. Ask whether the rhythm is fast or slow, and whether it is regular or irregular. It is helpful to ask the patient to tap the rhythm on a table top. This may provide clues to the underlying arrhythmia.

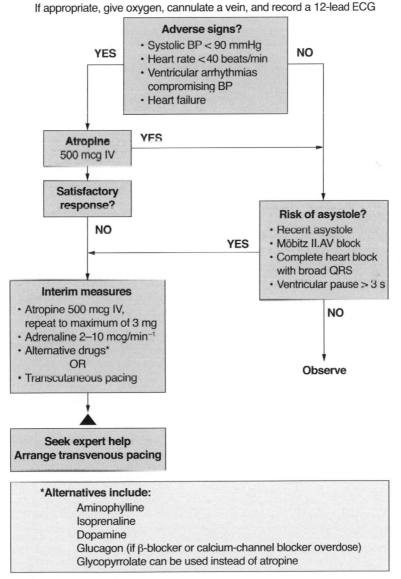

Figure 10.2 Algorithm for the management of bradycardia. Reproduced with kind permission of the Resuscitation Council (UK).

- Exacerbating factors. Sinus tachycardia on assuming the upright position is characteristic of postural orthostatic tachycardia syndrome. Palpitations associated with particular situations may occur in patients with phobic or panic disorders.
- A regular pounding sensation in the neck is characteristic of atrioventricular nodal re-entry tachycardia. It is caused by simultaneous contraction of the atria and ventricles so that the atria contract against closed atrioventricular valves, resulting in regular cannon waves.[2]
- Polyuria may occur during and following a supraventricular tachycardia, due to the release of atrial natriuretic peptide and the inhibition of ADH release, mediated by atrial stretch receptors.[3]

➤ Ask specifically about pre-syncope, syncope or chest pain occurring in conjunction with the palpitations. This suggests a paroxysmal cardiac arrhythmia that is causing cardiovascular compromise, and therefore demands more urgent investigation.
➤ Drug history. Theophyllines and sympathomimetics may cause palpitation.
➤ Alcohol and caffeine intake should be documented, and enquiry made about illicit drug use.
➤ A family history of cardiac arrhythmias or sudden cardiac death suggests a hereditary electrophysiological abnormality.

EXAMINATION
➤ Note the pulse rate, rhythm and volume.
➤ Check the blood pressure. Hypotension in conjunction with a tachy- or bradyarrhythmia suggests that the arrhythmia is causing cardiovascular compromise and requires urgent treatment. Hypertension in combination with sinus tachycardia suggests sympathetic overactivity.
➤ Check for clinical features of cardiac failure, including hypoxia, raised JVP, peripheral oedema, bilateral basal lung crackles or pleural effusions, and an S3 gallop rhythm. An arrhythmia that is causing cardiac failure demands urgent treatment.
➤ Look for clinical features associated with hyperthyroidism, such as anxiety, postural tremor, tachycardia, increased sweating, flushed skin or goitre. Ophthalmic abnormalities may include lid lag, lid retraction, chemosis, ophthalmoplegia and proptosis.
➤ Auscultate the heart, checking in particular for the early diastolic murmur of aortic regurgitation.

INVESTIGATIONS
The following core investigations are commonly required:
➤ Blood tests:
  - FBC (anaemia is a possible cause of palpitation)
  - U&Es, calcium and magnesium (electrolyte abnormalities may cause cardiac arrhythmias)
  - glucose.
➤ TFTs.
➤ Resting ECG.
➤ Ambulatory ECG monitor.

The following further investigations may be required:
➤ Echocardiogram. This may be required to rule out structural heart disease as an underlying cause of a cardiac arrhythmia, or to demonstrate aortic regurgitation.
➤ Cardiac electrophysiological studies.
➤ Tilt-table testing may be used to diagnose postural orthostatic tachycardia syndrome.
➤ A toxicology screen, focusing on cocaine, amphetamines and MDMA, may be required if illicit drug use is suspected.
➤ Twenty-four-hour urine collection for 5-HIAA (levels of which are raised in carcinoid syndrome) or catecholamines and VMA (levels of which are raised in phaeochromocytoma).
➤ ABG with carboxyhaemoglobin measurement should be performed if carbon monoxide poisoning is suspected.

REFERENCES
1 Resuscitation Council (UK). *Resuscitation Guidelines 2005*. London: Resuscitation Council (UK); 2005.
2 Gursoy S, Steurer G, Brugada J *et al.* The hemodynamic mechanism of pounding in the neck in atrioventricular nodal re-entrant tachycardia. *N Engl J Med*. 1992; **327**: 772–4.
3 Fujii T, Kojima S, Imanishi M *et al.* Different mechanisms of polyuria and natriuresis associated with paroxysmal supraventricular tachycardia. *Am J Cardiol*. 1991; **68**: 343–8.

CHAPTER 11

Oedema

PATHOPHYSIOLOGY AND AETIOLOGY

The body of a person who weighs 70 kg contains approximately 42 litres of fluid. This consists of around 28 litres of intracellular fluid and 14 litres of extracellular fluid.[1] The 14 litres of extracellular fluid in turn consist of approximately 3 litres of plasma, which lies within the circulation, and 11 litres of interstitial fluid, which surrounds the cells of the various body tissues. The distribution of fluid within the various body compartments under normal circumstances is shown in Figure 11.1. Oedema may be defined as an increase in interstitial fluid volume that is sufficient to cause clinically apparent swelling of soft tissue.

The volume of the extracellular compartment is determined mainly by the total body sodium content, and to a lesser extent by the total body water content. Sodium ions are kept almost exclusively within the extracellular compartment by Na^+/K^+ ATPase pumps on cell surface membranes. As water crosses cell membranes freely, an increase in total body sodium levels will result in an expansion of the extracellular compartment, due to the passive movement of water down the resulting osmotic gradient.

As mentioned above, the extracellular compartment consists of approximately 3 litres of plasma and 11 litres of interstitial fluid. This situation is maintained by two main mechanisms that act to keep fluid within the circulation. First, the capillary membranes are impermeable to a number of solutes, such as plasma proteins, thus trapping them within the circulation, where they exert an osmotic force. This is known as the oncotic pressure of the plasma. Secondly, the lymphatic system acts to drain excess interstitial fluid back into the circulation. These mechanisms may be disrupted by a number of factors, resulting in excess interstitial fluid and oedema. Some of these factors cause generalised oedema, whereas others cause localised oedema, as described below.

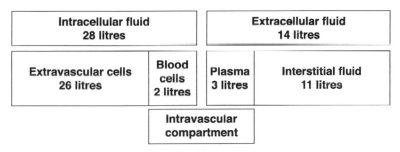

Figure 11.1 Fluid compartments in a person with a body weight of 70 kg.

Factors that cause generalised oedema

➤ **Increased capillary bed pressure.** This may result from increased pressure within the systemic veins (as occurs with cardiac failure), from an increased circulating volume (as may occur with chronic renal failure) or from arteriolar vasodilatation (as occurs in patients taking dihydropyridine calcium-channel antagonists). Increased capillary bed pressure will force more fluid into the interstitium, thus causing oedema.

➤ **Increased capillary permeability.** This usually results from the release of inflammatory mediators (e.g. in patients with sepsis). These have the effect of making capillaries more 'leaky', thus allowing plasma proteins to leak into the interstitium, drawing water with them by osmosis.

➤ **Reduced intravascular oncotic pressure.** Hypoalbuminaemia of any cause will reduce the body's ability to hold fluid within the circulation, thus causing leakage into the interstitium.

Each of the factors that cause generalised oedema will result in loss of fluid from the circulation into the interstitium. If this leaves the effective circulating volume depleted, the renin–angiotensin system will be activated, causing further salt and water retention and thus extracellular volume expansion, further worsening the oedema.

Factors that cause localised oedema
➤ **Venous obstruction or insufficiency.** This results in a local increase in capillary bed pressure due to increased pressure within the occluded draining veins, resulting in fluid transit from the circulation into the interstitium.
➤ **Lymphatic obstruction or insufficiency.** Disruption of the lymphatic system results in oedema by removing one of the main physiological mechanisms for returning interstitial fluid to the circulation.
The causes of oedema are listed in Table 11.1, with common causes highlighted in bold type.

EMERGENCY MANAGEMENT
➤ Ensure that airway, breathing and circulation are intact.
➤ Specific treatment will depend on the underlying diagnosis.

HISTORY
➤ Ask about the time course of the symptoms, and note the distribution of the oedema, in particular whether it is generalised or localised, and whether it is symmetrical or asymmetrical.
➤ Enquire about risk factors for venous thromboembolism. These include recent immobility, malignancy, current or recent pregnancy, personal or family history of venous thromboembolism, smoking, and use of the combined oral contraceptive pill.
➤ Associated symptoms may provide diagnostic clues.
  – Shortness of breath, orthopnoea or paroxysmal nocturnal dyspnoea suggest cardiac failure.
  – Anuria and oliguria are signs of renal failure.
  – Localised erythema or tenderness occurs with deep vein thrombosis.
  – Diarrhoea or steatorrhoea suggests malabsorption with hypoalbuminaemia.
  – Frothy urine occurs with severe proteinuria.
  – Urticaria or a skin rash may occur with hypersensitivity and complement-mediated reactions such as anaphylaxis.
➤ Past medical history. In particular, note any chronic cardiac, renal or hepatic conditions.
➤ Drug history. Dihydropyridine calcium-channel antagonists and fludrocortisone may cause oedema.

EXAMINATION
➤ General examination. Observe the patient's nutritional status, and any signs of chronic liver disease (e.g. jaundice, spider naevi or gynaecomastia). Urticaria or a skin rash suggests a hypersensitivity reaction or complement-mediated process. Lymphadenopathy may be due to malignant infiltration, which is a possible cause of lymphoedema.
➤ Observe the distribution of the oedema, and whether it is pitting or non-pitting. Non-pitting oedema is most likely to be chronic (e.g. due to lymphoedema).
➤ Assess the jugular venous pressure (JVP). A raised JVP occurs with cardiac failure, pericardial constriction, restrictive cardiomyopathy, cor pulmonale or primary pulmonary hypertension. Kussmaul's sign is present when the JVP rises on inspiration instead of falling. It occurs with pericardial constriction and restrictive cardiomyopathy.
➤ Palpate the precordium. A laterally displaced apex beat suggests cardiac failure, whereas a right ventricular (left parasternal) heave or palpable pulmonary second heart sound indicates cor pulmonale (very common) or primary pulmonary hypertension (rare).
➤ Auscultate the heart. An S_3 gallop rhythm may be audible with cardiac failure, whereas a prominent pulmonary second heart sound is associated with cor pulmonale or primary pulmonary hypertension.
➤ Examine the chest. A hyper-expanded chest with a prolonged expiratory phase and pursed lip breathing suggests chronic obstructive pulmonary disease with cor pulmonale. Bilateral basal crackles or pleural effusions occur with cardiac failure.
➤ Examine the abdomen. Ascites and hepatomegaly may occur with liver cirrhosis, cardiac failure, pericardial constriction, restrictive cardiomyopathy, cor pulmonale or primary pulmonary hypertension. Liver cirrhosis may also cause splenomegaly.

INVESTIGATIONS
The following core investigations are commonly required:
➤ Urine dip. Proteinuria occurs with nephrotic syndrome and pre-eclampsia. This may be further quantified by means of a 24-hour urine collection. The combination of haematuria and proteinuria suggests the possibility of glomerulonephritis.
➤ Blood tests:
  – FBC. Anaemia may occur with renal failure or liver cirrhosis.
  – U&Es and LFTs. Renal or hepatic failure may cause oedema.
  – CRP. This is raised with infection or inflammation.
  – Albumin. Hypoalbuminaemia may contribute to oedema.
  – D-dimer. This should be performed if deep vein thrombosis is suspected clinically.

Table 11.1 Causes of oedema

Generalised oedema			Localised oedema	
Increased capillary bed pressure	*Increased capillary permeability*	*Reduced intravascular oncotic pressure*	*Venous obstruction or insufficiency*	*Lymphatic obstruction or insufficiency*
Systemic venous hypertension ▲ Cardiac failure ▲ Cor pulmonale ▲ Restrictive cardiomyopathy ▲ Pericardial constriction ▲ Primary pulmonary hypertension Increased circulating volume ▲ Renal failure ▲ Liver cirrhosis ▲ Pregnancy ▲ Cushing's syndrome ▲ Exogenous mineralocorticoids ▲ Refeeding syndrome Arteriolar vasodilatation ▲ Dihydropyridine calcium channel antagonists	Systemic inflammatory response syndrome ▲ Sepsis ▲ Toxic shock syndrome ▲ Pancreatitis ▲ Trauma ▲ Burns Hypersensitivity or complement-mediated ▲ Anaphylaxis or anaphylactoid reaction ▲ Angioedema ▲ Mastocytosis ▲ Serum sickness Connective tissue disease ▲ RS3PE syndrome ▲ Polymyalgia rheumatica ▲ Undifferentiated spondyloarthropathy[2] ▲ POEMS syndrome ▲ Miscellaneous Miscellaneous ▲ Pre-eclampsia ▲ AILD ▲ Eosinophilia–myalgia syndrome	Nephrotic syndrome Hepatic failure Sepsis Malabsorption Protein-losing enteropathy Malnutrition	Deep vein thrombosis Chronic venous insufficiency Superior or inferior vena cava obstruction Congenital vascular abnormalities	Neoplasia ▲ Malignant infiltration ▲ Lymphoma ▲ Neurofibromatosis Trauma ▲ Surgery ▲ Radiotherapy ▲ Mechanical trauma Miscellaneous ▲ Sarcoidosis ▲ Yellow nail syndrome ▲ Ilioinguinal node sclerosis ▲ Lymphatic filariasis ▲ Podoconiosis ▲ Primary lymphoedema

➤ ECG. This may show left ventricular hypertrophy, suggesting cardiac failure.
➤ CXR. Cardiomegaly, pulmonary venous congestion or frank pulmonary oedema are features of cardiac failure.

The following further investigations may be required:
➤ Echocardiogram. This may reveal cardiac failure, pericardial constriction, restrictive cardiomyopathy or pulmonary hypertension.
➤ Venous leg Doppler. This is used to diagnose deep vein thrombosis.
➤ Abdominal USS. This may confirm the presence of ascites or liver cirrhosis. Alternatively, an intra-abdominal mass causing obstruction to lower limb venous return may be visualised.
➤ Lymphoscintigraphy. This is used to diagnose lymphatic obstruction.
➤ OGD with small bowel biopsy. This may reveal malabsorption or protein-losing enteropathy.
➤ Blood tests:
  – Complement components. These are abnormal in hereditary angioedema (HAE). The precise pattern of abnormality depends on the specific type of HAE (I, II or III).
  – Mast cell tryptase. This is raised following an anaphylactic reaction.
  – Serum electrophoresis. Monoclonal gammopathy occurs with POEMS syndrome.
  – Tissue transglutaminase or anti-endomysial/antigliadin antibodies. These occur in coeliac disease.

REFERENCES
1   Guyton AC, Hall JE. *Textbook of Medical Physiology*. 11th edn. Philadelphia, PA: Elsevier Saunders; 2006. pp. 292–3.
2   Olivieri I, Salvarani C, Cantini F *et al*. Ankylosing spondylitis and undifferentiated spondyloarthropathies: a clinical review and description of a disease subset with older age at onset. *Curr Opin Rheumatol*. 2001; **13**: 280–4.

CHAPTER 12

Limb pain

PATHOPHYSIOLOGY AND AETIOLOGY

Acute limb pain is most commonly caused by arterial occlusion, deep vein thrombosis or cellulitis. A subacute or chronic course may be caused by chronic arterial or venous insufficiency, but may also result from metabolic bone disease, malignant bone infiltration or neuropathy. The mechanisms of limb pain may be summarised as follows:

➤ impaired arterial blood supply
➤ impaired venous drainage
➤ infection, inflammation or trauma
➤ metabolic muscle or bone disease
➤ neoplasia
➤ neuropathy.

The causes of limb pain are listed in Table 12.1, with common causes highlighted in bold type.

EMERGENCY TREATMENT

➤ Check carefully for signs of acute limb ischaemia. If these are present, refer the patient promptly for a vascular surgical opinion, as early surgical intervention may be limb-saving.
➤ Think of deep vein thrombosis in a unilaterally swollen leg. If in doubt, treat with heparin until definitive investigations can be performed, unless contraindicated.
➤ A cellulitic-looking leg with pain and/or systemic illness that is out of proportion to the clinical features should prompt consideration of more serious infections such as necrotising fasciitis, and referral for an orthopaedic opinion. Urgent surgical debridement may be required.
➤ Consider compartment syndrome if a limb (usually a leg) that has recently undergone trauma or fracture develops disproportionate pain and/or symptoms and signs of ischaemia, such as paraesthesia, pallor, absent pulses, paralysis and cold peripheries. If this condition is suspected, any plaster cast should be immediately removed, and the patient referred to the orthopaedic surgeons for consideration of fasciotomy.

HISTORY

➤ Characteristics of the pain:
  – Time course of the symptoms. Acute limb ischaemia, deep vein thrombosis and soft tissue infection develop over a period of hours to days, whereas osteomyelitis and malignant bone infiltration run a more chronic course.
  – Distribution of pain.
  – Character of pain. Nerve root impingement may cause a characteristic shooting pain.
  – Exacerbating factors. Raynaud's syndrome is usually triggered by cold weather. Exercise-induced limb pain may be caused by both peripheral arterial insufficiency and spinal canal stenosis, in which case it is referred to as vascular and neurogenic claudication, respectively.
➤ Associated symptoms:
  – Leg swelling or erythema may be caused by deep vein thrombosis or soft tissue infection.
  – Pallor, paraesthesia and paralysis are symptoms of acute limb ischaemia.
  – Back pain, weakness or sensory changes suggest a neuropathic origin to the pain.
➤ Ask about risk factors for venous thromboembolism. These include recent immobility, malignancy, current or recent pregnancy, previous venous thromboembolism, smoking, and use of the combined oral contraceptive pill.

EXAMINATION

➤ Palpate the peripheral pulses (femoral, popliteal, dorsalis pedis and posterior tibial).
➤ Check for symptoms and signs of acute limb ischaemia, which can be remembered as the 'six Ps' (Pain, Paraesthesiae, Pallor, Pulselessness, Paralysis and Perishingly cold). Similar features may occur with compartment syndrome, in conjunction with tense shiny skin overlying the affected compartment.
➤ Further signs of peripheral vascular disease include prolonged capillary refill time, dependent rubor and a positive Buerger's test (pallor of the foot caused by elevation of the lower limb to 45°).
➤ Erythema or swelling of the leg suggests deep vein thrombosis or soft tissue infection.
➤ Weakness or sensory loss may be caused by acute limb ischaemia or spinal root compression.

Table 12.1 Causes of limb pain

Vascular disease	*Soft tissue disease*	*Bone disease*	*Neuropathy*
Arterial occlusion	Mechanical factors	Fracture	Spinal root compression
➤ Arterial thromboembolism	➤ Trauma		➤ Spondylosis
➤ Peripheral vascular disease	➤ Haematoma	Osteomyelitis	➤ Spondylolisthesis
➤ Buerger's disease	➤ Ruptured Baker's cyst	➤ Bacterial	➤ Vertebral fracture
➤ Arterial trauma	➤ Compartment syndrome	➤ Tuberculous	➤ Prolapsed intervertebral disc
➤ Takayasu arteritis		➤ Fungal	➤ Spinal canal tumour
➤ Giant-cell arteritis	Metabolic myopathies	➤ Echinococcal	➤ Spinal abscess
➤ Kawasaki disease	➤ Alcoholic myopathy		➤ Miscellaneous
	➤ Drug-induced myopathy	Metabolic bone disease	
Small vessel disease	➤ Rhabdomyolysis	➤ Osteomalacia	Peripheral neuropathy
➤ Raynaud's syndrome	➤ Hypothyroidism	➤ Renal osteodystrophy	➤ Compression neuropathy
➤ Sickle-cell crisis	➤ Carnitine palmitoyltransferase deficiency	➤ Paget's disease	➤ Diabetic amyotrophy
➤ Erythromelalgia		➤ Hyperparathyroidism	➤ Neuralgic amyotrophy
➤ Cold agglutinin disease	➤ Glycogen storage diseases	➤ Scurvy	➤ Idiopathic lumbosacral plexus neuropathy
➤ Decompression sickness		➤ Vitamin A toxicity	➤ Shingles
	Soft tissue infection		➤ Post-herpetic neuralgia
Venous occlusion	➤ Cellulitis	Bone infiltration or inflammation	➤ Reflex sympathetic dystrophy
➤ Deep vein thrombosis	➤ Pyomyositis	➤ Metastatic malignancy	➤ Fabry's disease
➤ Superficial thrombophlebitis	➤ Necrotising fasciitis	➤ Multiple myeloma	➤ Miscellaneous
➤ Chronic venous insufficiency	➤ Gas gangrene	➤ Leukaemia	
➤ Inferior or superior vena cava obstruction		➤ Lymphoma	Syringomyelia
	Infectious myositis	➤ Mastocytosis	
	➤ HIV	➤ Myelofibrosis	Thalamic pain syndrome
	➤ HTLV-1	➤ Polycythaemia vera	
	➤ Influenza	➤ Thalassaemia	Fibromyalgia
	➤ Enteroviruses	➤ Langerhans cell histiocytosis	
	➤ Lyme disease	➤ Erdheim-Chester disease	
	➤ Tuberculosis	➤ Schnitzler syndrome	
	➤ Toxoplasmosis	➤ Primary bone tumour	
	➤ Chagas' disease	➤ Gaucher's disease	
	➤ Trichinosis	➤ Chronic recurrent multifocal osteomyelitis	
	➤ Cysticercosis		
	➤ Miscellaneous		
	Inflammation		
	➤ Eosinophilia-myalgia syndrome		
	➤ Eosinophilic fasciitis		
	➤ Fibrodysplasia ossificans progressiva		
	➤ Focal myositis		
	➤ Macrophagic myofasciitis		
	Muscle tumour		
	Muscle cramp		

INVESTIGATIONS

The following core investigations are commonly required:
➤ Blood tests:
  – Raised WBC and CRP are signs of infection.
  – D-dimer is raised with deep vein thrombosis.
➤ Arterial Doppler may reveal arterial thromboembolism or chronic arterial insufficiency
➤ Venous Doppler is used to diagnose deep vein thrombosis.

The following further investigations may be required:
➤ Arterial angiogram. This is used for the diagnosis and treatment of acute arterial occlusion.
➤ Plain limb radiology. This may show evidence of osteomyelitis, multiple myeloma or other malignant infiltrations.
➤ Limb MRI. Musculoskeletal injuries, infections or tumours may be visualised.
➤ Spine X-ray or MRI. These should be requested if spinal root compression is suspected.

CHAPTER 13

Abdominal pain

PATHOPHYSIOLOGY AND AETIOLOGY

Abdominal pain may be classified as visceral, somatic or neuropathic. Visceral abdominal pain arises from the solid and hollow internal organs, and is characteristically dull and poorly localised. It is mediated by slow-conducting C fibres. Visceral pain may be caused by distension of a hollow organ, contraction of a muscular organ against an obstruction, distension of the capsule enclosing a solid organ, irritation of the mucosa lining the inside of a hollow organ, or ischaemia of a hollow or solid organ. Somatic pain is caused by peritoneal irritation or by injury to musculoskeletal or cutaneous structures. It is characteristically sharp and well localised to the site of pathology, and is mediated by fast-conducting A-delta fibres. Neuropathic pain arises from damage to the brain, spinal cord, nerve roots or peripheral nerves, and may have a variety of qualities. The distribution of pain may suggest the site of the lesion.

Some conditions may cause abdominal pain by more than one mechanism. For example, acute appendicitis classically causes periumbilical visceral pain initially, due to obstruction of the appendix. This is followed some hours later by somatic pain localised to the right iliac fossa, caused by inflammation of the appendix and thus peritoneal irritation.

The causes of abdominal pain are listed in Table 13.1, with common causes highlighted in bold type.

EMERGENCY MANAGEMENT

➤ Provide fluid resuscitation if there is evidence of shock, sepsis or hypovolaemia. One exception is the patient with ruptured abdominal aortic aneurysm, in whom a degree of hypotension should be tolerated in order to avoid disrupting a partially formed thrombus and causing torrential bleeding.
➤ The initial priority is to diagnose or rule out causes of abdominal pain that require urgent surgical treatment, such as acute appendicitis and ruptured ectopic pregnancy.
➤ Provide adequate analgesia. This should not be withheld due to fear that it would 'mask' the diagnosis.

HISTORY

➤ Time course and speed of onset of pain.
➤ Site of pain. Although wide variations occur, the location of the pain may suggest the organ that is most likely to be involved:
  – epigastric region: oesophagus, stomach, duodenum or pancreas
  – right hypochondrium: liver or biliary tract
  – left hypochondrium: stomach or spleen
  – umbilical region: small bowel, proximal colon or testicle
  – right or left flank: kidney or ureter
  – suprapubic region: distal colon, bladder, cervix or uterus
  – right iliac fossa: appendix, Meckel's diverticulum, caecum, ovary
  – left iliac fossa: sigmoid colon, ovary.
➤ Radiation or associated pain:
  – Radiation to the back may occur with abdominal aortic aneurysm, renal or ureteric disease and pancreatic disease, as well as with a posterior duodenal ulcer or inflammation of a retrocaecal appendix.
  – Chest pain may occur with myocardial infarction, pleural irritation or pericardial irritation.

Table 13.1 Causes of abdominal pain

Gastrointestinal

Perforated viscus

Colonic inflammation
- Appendicitis
- Diverticulitis
- Inflammatory bowel disease
- Neutropenic colitis

Small bowel inflammation
- Meckel's diverticulitis
- Crohn's disease
- Eosinophilic gastroenteritis
- Hypereosinophilic syndrome
- Radiation enteritis
- Graft-versus-host disease
- Idiopathic ulcerative enteritis

Gastric or oesophageal inflammation
- Oesophagitis
- Gastritis
- GORD
- Peptic ulcer disease

Bowel obstruction
- Incarcerated hernia
- Adhesions
- Stricture
- Volvulus
- Tumour
- Intussusception
- Gallstone ileus
- Sclerosing peritonitis

Infection
- Viral gastroenteritis
- Bacterial gastroenteritis
- Pseudomembranous colitis
- Phlegmonous gastritis
- Phlegmonous enteritis or colitis
- Yersiniosis
- Tuberculosis
- Typhoid fever
- Brucellosis
- Tularaemia
- Fungal infection
- Protozoan infection
- Helminth infection
- Miscellaneous

Vascular insufficiency
- Acute mesenteric ischaemia
- Mesenteric angina

Small vessel vasculopathy
- Henoch–Schönlein purpura
- Polyarteritis nodosa
- Microscopic polyangiitis
- Churg–Strauss syndrome
- Behçet's disease
- Cryoglobulinaemia
- Systemic lupus erythematosus
- TTP/HUS
- Cholesterol embolism
- Degos' disease
- Decompression sickness
- Miscellaneous

Hepatobiliary and pancreatic

Pancreatic
- Acute pancreatitis
- Chronic pancreatitis
- Pancreatic cancer

Biliary
- Biliary colic
- Acute cholecystitis
- Acute cholangitis
- Cholangiocarcinoma
- Primary sclerosing cholangitis
- Sphincter of Oddi dysfunction
- Biliary peritonitis

Hepatic
- Viral hepatitis
- Alcoholic hepatitis
- Autoimmune hepatitis
- Toxic liver injury
- Hepatic abscess
- Fitz–Hugh–Curtis syndrome
- Hepatic congestion
- Hepatic infarction
- Pre-eclampsia
- HELLP syndrome
- Acute fatty liver of pregnancy
- Spontaneous hepatic rupture
- Hepatic tumour
- Hepatic artery aneurysm

Genitourinary and gynaecological

Urinary tract obstruction
- Bladder outflow obstruction
- Ureteric colic
- Nephrolithiasis

Urinary tract infection
- Cystitis
- Pyelonephritis
- Perinephric abscess
- Renal abcess
- Tuberculosis
- Miscellaneous

Renal conditions
- Renal infarction
- Renal cyst haemorrhage
- Renal cell carcinoma
- Glomerulonephritis
- Acute interstitial nephritis
- Transplant rejection
- Loin pain haematuria syndrome

Testicular and prostatic disorders
- Torsion of testis
- Epididymitis
- Orchitis
- Prostatitis

Pelvic inflammatory disease
- Bacterial
- Tuberculous

Ovarian pathology
- Ovarian torsion
- Ruptured ovarian cyst
- Ovarian cancer
- OHSS
- Mumps

Miscellaneous local conditions

Intra-abdominal
- Haemorrhage
- Peritonitis
- Abscess
- Tumour
- Massive organomegaly
- Mesenteric adenitis
- Aortic aneurysm
- Aortic dissection
- Sickle-cell crisis
- Splenic infarction
- Splenic rupture
- Omental torsion or infarction

Thoracic
- Myocardial infarction
- Pneumonia
- Empyema
- Pneumothorax
- Pulmonary infarction
- Pericarditis

Musculoskeletal
- Rectus sheath haematoma
- Muscle tear
- Osteitis pubis
- Bornholm disease

Neuropathic
- Shingles
- Post-herpetic neuralgia
- Peripheral nerve compression
- Spinal root irritation
- Transverse myelitis
- Tabes dorsalis
- Abdominal epilepsy

Systemic conditions

Endocrine/metabolic
- Hypercalcaemia
- Diabetic ketoacidosis
- Hypoglycaemia
- Lactic acidosis
- Acute porphyria
- Adrenal insufficiency
- Hyperthyroidism[2]
- Phaeochromocytoma

Poisoning
- Food poisoning
- Botulism
- Carbon monoxide
- Heavy metals
- Organophosphates
- Miscellaneous

Systemic infection
- Toxic shock syndrome
- Dengue fever
- Viral haemorrhagic fever
- Rickettsiosis
- Malaria
- Babesiosis
- Miscellaneous

Familial periodic fevers
- Familial Mediterranean fever
- TRAPS
- HIDS

Miscellaneous
- Opiate withdrawal
- TINU syndrome[3]
- Acute glaucoma[4]

Gastrointestinal	Hepatobiliary and pancreatic	Genitourinary and gynaecological	Miscellaneous local conditions	Systemic conditions
▲ Retroperitoneal fibrosis ▲ Superior mesenteric artery syndrome ▲ Cronkhite–Canada syndrome ▲ Hereditary angioedema ▲ Mastocytosis ▲ Anaphylaxis Neoplasia ▲ **Oesophagus** ▲ **Stomach** ▲ Small bowel ▲ Colon or rectum Functional ▲ **Constipation** ▲ Irritable bowel syndrome Structural disorders ▲ Mallory–Weiss tear ▲ Oesophageal rupture ▲ Intramural haemorrhage ▲ Pneumatosis intestinalis Bowel dysmotility ▲ Ogilvie's syndrome ▲ Chagas' disease ▲ Fabry's disease ▲ Familial visceral myopathy ▲ Acute intravascular haemolysis[1] ▲ Miscellaneous		Endometriosis Uterine fibroid Complications of pregnancy ▲ **Miscarriage** ▲ Ectopic pregnancy ▲ Placental abruption ▲ Puerperal fever ▲ Uterine rupture		

- Right shoulder tip pain occurs with any pathology that irritates the right hemidiaphragm. Examples include subphrenic abscess and Fitz–Hugh–Curtis syndrome.
- Left shoulder tip pain occurs with any pathology that irritates the left hemidiaphragm. Examples include splenic abscess and splenic rupture.

➤ Character and severity of pain:
- Visceral pain is dull in character and poorly localised. Patients often move around in an attempt to find a comfortable position. If it is caused by the intermittent contraction of a hollow organ against an obstruction (e.g. in small bowel obstruction or ureteric calculi), the pain will be episodic or colicky.
- Somatic pain is sharp in character and well localised. Patients are often unwilling to move or cough, as this exacerbates the pain.
- Neuropathic pain is variable in character. For instance, the pain of shingles is constant and may be described as 'burning', whereas spinal root irritation often produces shooting pain that is worse on movement. The distribution of pain may suggest the site of pathology.

➤ Exacerbating and relieving factors:
- Peritoneal irritation is exacerbated by movement or coughing.
- The pain of pancreatitis may be relieved by sitting forward.

➤ Associated symptoms:
- Fever suggests infection or inflammation.
- Rigors occur with infection, particularly pyelonephritis and acute cholangitis.
- Nausea and vomiting may occur with a variety of conditions, particularly those that cause distension of a hollow organ or irritation of the gastrointestinal tract.
- Haematemesis or melaena may be caused by peptic ulcer disease or gastritis.
- Rectal bleeding occurs with ulcerative colitis and ischaemic colitis.
- Diarrhoea most commonly occurs with infection, inflammation or ischaemia of the colon.
- Constipation may cause abdominal pain if severe. Absolute constipation, with absent passage of both stool and flatus, suggests bowel obstruction.
- Abdominal distension is a feature of bowel obstruction.
- Jaundice occurs with hepatobiliary or pancreatic disease.
- Frequency of micturition, dysuria and haematuria are features of urinary tract disease.
- Scrotal swelling occurs with testicular disorders.
- Vaginal discharge suggests pelvic inflammatory disease.
- Abnormal vaginal bleeding may occur with ectopic pregnancy, placental abruption, miscarriage or gynaecological malignancy.
- Localised rash may occur with shingles, whereas generalised rash suggests systemic infection, vasculitis or connective tissue disease.
- Joint pain or swelling may occur with systemic vasculitis, connective tissue disease, familial periodic fevers and some systemic infections.

➤ Menstrual history:
- Ask about the normal cycle length and regularity.
- Ascertain the date of the last menstrual period. A late or missed period may be a feature of ectopic pregnancy.

➤ Enquire about any family history of hereditary angioedema or familial periodic fevers if relevant.
➤ Ask about alcohol intake and recent foreign travel.

EXAMINATION

➤ Check for signs of hypovolaemic or septic shock. These include hypotension, a postural drop in blood pressure, tachycardia, tachypnoea, reduced urine output and confusion. Cool peripheries, prolonged capillary refill time and a weak thready pulse occur in hypovolaemia and late sepsis, whereas warm peripheries and a bounding pulse occur in early sepsis. Hypovolaemia may be due to intra-abdominal haemorrhage (e.g. from an abdominal aortic aneurysm, or from third space losses into an obstructed bowel), whereas sepsis may have a systemic or intra-abdominal source.

➤ General examination:
- Pyrexia suggests infection or inflammation.
- Observe the demeanour of the patient. Are they well or unwell? Is the pain mild or severe? Are they lying still (somatic pain) or moving about and restless (visceral pain)?
- Jaundice suggests hepatobiliary or pancreatic disease.
- Note the presence of any rash. Is it localised, in a dermatomal distribution (shingles) or generalised (systemic infection, vasculitis or connective tissue disease)?
- Lymphadenopathy may occur with gastrointestinal malignancy and some systemic infections.
- Anaemia occurs with gastrointestinal or intra-abdominal haemorrhage.
- Skin crease or mucous membrane pigmentation suggests primary adrenal insufficiency, whereas ketotic breath is a feature of diabetic ketoacidosis.

➤ Abdominal examination:
- Note any abdominal distension or a visible mass.

- Visible peristalsis suggests bowel obstruction.
- Bruising in the periumbilical region (Cullen's sign) or flank (Grey–Turner's sign) suggests acute pancreatitis.
- Note the location and severity of any abdominal tenderness.
- Signs of peritonism include guarding, rigidity, rebound tenderness and percussion tenderness.
- Abdominal wall tenderness test. Tensing the abdominal wall muscles by lifting the head and shoulders off the bed will exacerbate tenderness caused by abdominal wall pathology, but will relieve tenderness caused by peritoneal pathology.
- Psoas sign. Pain upon hyperextending the right hip suggests psoas muscle irritation due to a nearby inflamed appendix.
- Obturator sign. Pain upon flexing and internally rotating the right hip suggests irritation of the obturator internus muscle due to a nearby inflamed appendix.
- Rovsing's sign. Right lower quadrant pain that is elicited by pressure in the left lower quadrant is a further sign of acute appendicitis.
- Murphy's sign. This is elicited by applying moderate pressure to the right hypochondrium and asking the patient to inspire deeply. In acute cholecystitis, the patient will stop breathing abruptly as the inflamed gallbladder moves down and meets the examiner's hand.
- Hepatomegaly, splenomegaly or other abdominal masses should be noted, and an abdominal aortic aneurysm should be specifically sought.
- The presence of ascites should be elicited by testing for shifting dullness or a fluid thrill.
- Bowel sounds are absent with peritonitis. High-pitched, active bowel sounds occur with bowel obstruction.
- Hernial orifices. An incarcerated hernia may cause bowel obstruction. A tender irreducible hernia suggests strangulation.
- Femoral pulses may be absent with aortic dissection or with bleeding aortic or iliac artery aneurysms.
- External genitalia. Scrotal swelling or tenderness may be detected.
- Rectal examination. An obstructing mass may be palpable. Rectal tenderness, especially on the right, may be present with pelvic appendicitis.
- Bimanual and speculum examination of the vagina is indicated if a gynaecological cause of the pain is suspected.
➤ Respiratory examination may reveal evidence of pneumonia, empyema or pneumothorax, which are possible causes of referred abdominal pain.

INVESTIGATIONS

The following core investigations are commonly required:
➤ Blood tests:
- Group and save should be sent in case urgent surgery is required.
- FBC. Anaemia suggests intra-abdominal haemorrhage.
- Clotting. This is deranged with hepatic failure.
- U&Es. Intra-abdominal sepsis may be complicated by acute kidney injury.
- LFTs. These may reveal a cholestatic or hepatitic pattern of abnormalities.
- Albumin. Levels are low with hepatic failure.
- Calcium. Hypercalcaemia may cause abdominal pain.
- CRP. This is raised with infection and inflammation.
- Amylase. Activity is raised with pancreatitis.
- Lactate. Levels are raised with severe sepsis or haemorrhage causing shock, and with bowel ischaemia.
➤ Urine dip:
- Haematuria may occur with urinary tract infection or calculi, as well as with acute appendicitis.
- Nitrites and leucocytes are a feature of urinary tract infection. Leucocytes may be seen with acute appendicitis.
- Glucose and ketones are seen with diabetic ketoacidosis.
➤ Pregnancy test.
➤ ECG may be diagnostic of myocardial infarction.
➤ Imaging.
- Erect CXR should be performed in order to detect subdiaphragmatic air, indicating perforation of a hollow organ. Pneumonia, empyema or pneumothorax may also be seen.
- Plain abdominal X-ray may reveal bowel obstruction, toxic bowel dilatation or constipation. Free intraperitoneal air is indicated by both the inner and outer aspect of the bowel wall being clearly visible (Rigler's sign).

The following further investigations may be required:
➤ Biochemistry:
- ABG may reveal metabolic acidosis in cases of septic or hypovolaemic shock, bowel ischaemia and diabetic ketoacidosis.

- Troponin I levels are raised from 12 hours after a myocardial infarction.
- Vasculitis and autoantibody screen. This should include ANA, ENA, anti-dsDNA (SLE), anti-SMA or anti-LKMA (autoimmune hepatitis), ANCA (Churg–Strauss syndrome) and cryoglobulins.
- C1 inhibitor, and C2 and C4 complement components may be low in hereditary angioedema.
- Urinary porphyrin levels are raised with acute intermittent porphyria.
➤ Microbiology:
  - blood culture
  - urine MC&S
  - stool culture and microscopy for ova and parasites
  - stool *Clostridium difficile* toxin test
  - microscopy and culture of urethral or vaginal discharge
  - high vaginal swab
  - hepatitis serology.
➤ Imaging:
  - Intravenous urogram. This may be required in order to diagnose renal tract calculi.
  - USS of the abdomen. Gallstone disease, renal tract calculi, bladder outflow obstruction, abdominal aortic aneurysm, ectopic pregnancy, intra-abdominal collection, ascites and abdominal wall haematoma may be readily diagnosed.
  - CT of the abdomen. Bowel obstruction, perforation or ischaemia, pancreatitis, intra-abdominal collection or haemorrhage, renal tract calculi, abdominal aortic aneurysm, tumours and a variety of other pathologies may be apparent.
  - OGD. This may allow visualisation of peptic ulcer disease, oesophagitis or gastritis.
  - Flexible sigmoidoscopy. This is helpful in the diagnosis of diverticulitis and inflammatory or infective colitis.
  - ERCP or MRCP. These are used for the diagnosis of biliary tract disease. Therapeutic interventions such as the removal of gallstones may be performed during ERCP.
  - Angiogram or MR angiogram. These allow diagnosis of mesenteric ischaemia, or thrombosis of the renal arteries, hepatic artery or portal vein.

REFERENCES
1 Rother RP, Bell L, Hillmen P *et al*. The clinical sequelae of intravascular haemolysis and extracellular plasma haemoglobin. *JAMA*. 2005; **293**: 1653–62.
2 Harper MB. Vomiting, nausea and abdominal pain: unrecognized symptoms of thyrotoxicosis. *J Fam Pract*. 1989; **29**(4): 382–6.
3 Goda C, Kotake S, Ichiishi A. Clinical features in tubulointerstitial nephritis and uveitis (TINU) syndrome. *Am J Ophthalmol*. 2005; **140**: 637–41.
4 Dayan M, Turner B, McGhee C. Lesson of the week: acute angle closure glaucoma masquerading as systemic illness. *BMJ*. 1996; **313**: 413–15.

CHAPTER 14

Nausea and vomiting

PATHOPHYSIOLOGY AND AETIOLOGY

Vomiting is the forcible expulsion of gastric contents from the mouth. It is often preceded by the unpleasant sensation of nausea. Vomiting is mediated by the emetic centre in the medulla, which receives afferent neurons from the gastrointestinal tract, the chemoreceptor trigger zone in the medulla, the vestibular apparatus and the cerebral cortex. There are six main stimuli that cause nausea or vomiting:

1   distension or obstruction of a hollow organ
2   exposure of the gastrointestinal mucosa to an irritant or toxic substance
3   stimulation of the chemoreceptor trigger zone
4   abnormal stimuli arising from the vestibular system
5   raised intracranial pressure
6   cerebral factors.

The causes of nausea and vomiting are listed in Table 14.1, with common causes highlighted in bold type.

EMERGENCY MANAGEMENT

➤   Ensure that the airway is patent. If the patient is unconscious, turn them into the left lateral position and use suction to remove vomitus from the mouth.
➤   Profuse vomiting may cause hypovolaemia. Fluid resuscitation with normal saline should be provided, with potassium replacement if required.

HISTORY

➤   Note the time course of symptoms and the frequency of vomiting.
➤   Note the appearance of the vomitus.
    –   Fresh blood or 'coffee-grounds' suggests upper gastrointestinal bleeding.
    –   Bilious vomiting occurs with small bowel obstruction.
    –   Faeculent vomiting suggests large bowel obstruction.
➤   Associated symptoms:
    –   Fever suggests infection.
    –   Weight loss occurs with gastrointestinal malignancy.
    –   Colicky abdominal pain is characteristic of bowel obstruction.
    –   Diarrhoea in association with vomiting suggests infective gastroenteritis or food poisoning.
    –   Melaena is clear evidence of upper gastrointestinal bleeding.
    –   Jaundice may be caused by choledocholithiasis, acute hepatitis, hepatic failure, HELLP syndrome or acute fatty liver of pregnancy.
    –   Headache should alert the clinician to the possibility of raised intracranial pressure or pre-eclampsia.
    –   Ataxia suggests cerebellar pathology, whereas vertigo occurs with vestibular system disease.
    –   Chest pain with vomiting may occur with myocardial infarction, whereas severe chest pain following a bout of vomiting may be due to oesophageal rupture.
➤   Dietary history. Note any recent dietary indiscretion such as eating undercooked meat. This would suggest food poisoning, particularly if others who ate the same food have developed similar symptoms.

EXAMINATION

➤   Assess the airway. Vomiting may cause aspiration with airway occlusion.
➤   Check the vital signs. These include temperature, pulse, blood pressure, respiratory rate and oxygen saturations.
➤   General examination:
    –   Check for signs of hypovolaemia. These include tachycardia, tachypnoea, hypotension or postural hypotension, oliguria, confusion, weak thready pulse, cool peripheries, prolonged capillary refill time, reduced skin turgor, dry mucous membranes and low JVP.
    –   Jaundice suggests biliary or hepatic pathology.
    –   Uraemic flap and hepatic flap occur with severe uraemia and hepatic encephalopathy, respectively.
    –   Ketotic breath may be detectable in patients with diabetic ketoacidosis.
    –   Skin crease or mucous membrane pigmentation occurs with primary adrenal insufficiency.
➤   Abdominal examination:

Table 14.1 Causes of nausea and vomiting

Distension or obstruction of a hollow organ	Gastrointestinal tract irritation	Chemoreceptor trigger zone stimulation	Vestibular system disorders	Raised intracranial pressure	Cerebral factors
Biliary obstruction ▲ Biliary colic ▲ Choledocholithiasis ▲ Acute cholecystitis ▲ Acute cholangitis Small bowel obstruction ▲ Incarcerated hernia ▲ Adhesions ▲ Stricture ▲ Tumour ▲ Intussusception ▲ Volvulus ▲ Gallstone ileus ▲ Sclerosing peritonitis ▲ Retroperitoneal fibrosis ▲ Superior mesenteric artery syndrome ▲ Intramural haematoma ▲ Cronkhite-Canada syndrome ▲ Hereditary angioedema ▲ Mastocytosis ▲ Anaphylaxis Gastric outflow obstruction ▲ Pyloric stenosis ▲ Gastric volvulus ▲ Antral web Large bowel obstruction ▲ Sigmoid volvulus ▲ Malignancy ▲ Acute appendicitis ▲ Toxic megacolon Dysmotility ▲ Peritonitis ▲ Ileus	Gastric mucosal irritation ▲ Upper gastrointestinal haemorrhage ▲ Peptic ulcer disease ▲ Food poisoning ▲ NSAIDs ▲ Alcohol ▲ Miscellaneous Infective gastroenteritis ▲ Viral ▲ Bacterial ▲ Fungal ▲ Protozoan ▲ Helminth Neoplasia ▲ Gastric cancer ▲ Gastric lymphoma ▲ Gastrointestinal stromal tumour Vascular insufficiency ▲ Acute mesenteric ischaemia ▲ Mesenteric angina Small vessel vasculopathy ▲ Henoch-Schönlein purpura ▲ Polyarteritis nodosa ▲ Microscopic polyangiitis ▲ Churg-Strauss syndrome ▲ Behçet's disease ▲ Cryoglobulinaemia ▲ Systemic lupus erythematosus ▲ TTP/HUS ▲ Cholesterol embolism	Metabolic and systemic disorders ▲ Sepsis ▲ Renal failure ▲ Hepatic failure ▲ Acute hepatitis ▲ Acute pancreatitis ▲ Diabetic ketoacidosis ▲ Hypercalcaemia ▲ Hyponatraemia ▲ Hypoglycaemia ▲ Acute porphyria ▲ Heat illness Complications of pregnancy ▲ Hyperemesis gravidarum ▲ Pre-eclampsia ▲ Eclampsia ▲ HELLP syndrome ▲ Acute fatty liver of pregnancy ▲ Ectopic pregnancy ▲ Hydatidiform mole Drugs and toxins ▲ Opiates ▲ Cytotoxic chemotherapy ▲ Erythromycin ▲ Heavy metals ▲ Miscellaneous	Motion sickness Vestibular or cochlear disease ▲ Vestibular neuritis ▲ Benign paroxysmal positional vertigo ▲ Ménière's disease ▲ Perilymph fistula ▲ Vestibular schwannoma ▲ Vestibular paroxysmia ▲ Labyrinthitis ▲ Miscellaneous Brainstem disease ▲ Thromboembolic stroke ▲ Haemorrhage ▲ Vertebral artery dissection ▲ Vertebrobasilar insufficiency ▲ Basilar migraine ▲ Multiple sclerosis ▲ Acute disseminated encephalomyelitis ▲ Paraneoplastic brainstem encephalitis ▲ Miscellaneous	Intracranial tumour Infection ▲ Meningitis ▲ Encephalitis ▲ Intracranial abscess ▲ Subdural empyema ▲ Tuberculoma ▲ Malaria ▲ African trypanosomiasis ▲ Toxoplasmosis ▲ Cysticercosis ▲ Hydatid disease ▲ Intracranial fungal infection ▲ Miscellaneous Intracranial haemorrhage ▲ Subarachnoid ▲ Subdural ▲ Extradural ▲ Intracerebral ▲ Cerebellar Ischaemia ▲ Cerebral infarction ▲ Cerebellar infarction ▲ Cerebral venous thrombosis Miscellaneous ▲ Acute mountain sickness ▲ Hydrocephalus ▲ Subdural hygroma ▲ Idiopathic intracranial hypertension ▲ Hypertensive encephalopathy ▲ PRES	Head injury Syncope Seizure Pain ▲ Migraine ▲ Myocardial infarction ▲ Ureteric colic ▲ Ovarian cyst torsion ▲ Testicular torsion ▲ Glaucoma ▲ Miscellaneous Psychological ▲ Bulimia nervosa ▲ Anorexia nervosa ▲ Functional

Distension or obstruction of a hollow organ	Gastrointestinal tract irritation	Chemoreceptor trigger zone stimulation	Vestibular system disorders	Raised intracranial pressure	Cerebral factors
▲ Gastroparesis	▲ Degos' disease				
▲ Autonomic neuropathy	▲ Decompression sickness				
▲ Ogilvie's syndrome	▲ Miscellaneous				
▲ Fabry's disease					
▲ Familial visceral myopathy[1]	Miscellaneous				
▲ Phaeochromocytoma[2]	▲ Eosinophilic gastroenteritis				
▲ Adrenal insufficiency[2]	▲ Hypereosinophilic syndrome				
▲ Hyperthyroidism[3]	▲ Haemophagocytic lymphohistiocytosis				
▲ Miscellaneous	▲ Radiation enteritis				
	▲ Graft-versus-host disease				
	▲ Idiopathic ulcerative enteritis				
	▲ Endometriosis				

- Severe abdominal tenderness or signs of peritonism such as guarding, rigidity, percussion tenderness and rebound tenderness suggests perforation of a viscus or bowel ischaemia. Urgent surgical review is indicated.
- Abdominal distension suggests small or large bowel obstruction or dysmotility.
- A palpable abdominal mass may be due to gastrointestinal malignancy.
- Auscultate the bowel sounds. Active bowel sounds occur with small bowel obstruction, whereas reduced or absent bowel sounds suggest generalised dysmotility.
- Perform a rectal examination. Melaena is a reliable sign of upper gastrointestinal haemorrhage. It should be noted that oral iron supplements also cause black stools, but these do not have the characteristic offensive smell of melaena.
➤ Neurological examination:
- Reduced level of consciousness may occur with raised intracranial pressure or severe metabolic disturbances.
- Focal neurological deficits occur with cerebral pathology such as thromboembolic stroke, haemorrhage, tumour and infection.
- Ataxia, reduced coordination and nystagmus suggest vestibular system or cerebellar disease.

INVESTIGATIONS
The following core investigations are commonly required:
➤ Blood tests:
- FBC. Anaemia may be due to gastrointestinal haemorrhage or malignancy.
- INR. Clotting abnormalities may result from hepatic failure.
- U&Es and calcium. Renal failure, hypercalcaemia and hyponatraemia are possible causes of nausea and vomiting.
- LFTs. These are likely to be abnormal with hepatic disorders such as HELLP syndrome.
- CRP. This is raised with infection and inflammation.
- Glucose. This is raised in diabetic ketoacidosis.
- Amylase. Activity of this enzyme is raised with pancreatitis.
➤ ABG. Diabetic ketoacidosis and renal failure cause metabolic acidosis, whereas vomiting itself may result in metabolic alkalosis.
➤ Urine dip and MC&S.
- Nitrites and leucocytes occur with urinary tract infection.
- Ketonuria and glycosuria are features of diabetic ketoacidosis.
- A pregnancy test should be performed in women of childbearing age.
➤ ECG should be performed to diagnose or rule out myocardial ischaemia.
➤ Imaging.
- Plain abdominal X-ray may reveal small or large bowel dilatation.
- Erect CXR may reveal subdiaphragmatic air, which suggests perforation of a viscus. Aspiration pneumonia secondary to vomiting may also be apparent.

The following further investigations may be required:
➤ Imaging:
- Abdominal USS or CT scan may reveal gallstones, renal calculi, gastrointestinal tumours or other intra-abdominal pathology.
- CT of the brain may visualise a thromboembolic stroke, intracranial haemorrhage, tumour or other space-occupying lesion.
- MRI of the brain is particularly useful for visualising brainstem or cerebellar lesions.
➤ Lumbar puncture. This should only be performed after raised intracranial pressure has been ruled out by CT of the head and fundoscopy.
- Xanthochromia is diagnostic of subarachnoid haemorrhage.
- Microscopy and culture may be diagnostic of bacterial meningitis.
- Staining for acid-fast bacilli and CSF mycobacterial culture should be performed if tuberculous meningitis is a possibility.
- India ink staining for cryptococcal meningitis should be performed if this condition is suspected.
- Meningococcal PCR.
- Herpes simplex virus PCR.
➤ Blood tests:
- Troponin I levels are raised from 12 hours after myocardial infarction.
- The short tetracosactide test may be diagnostic of adrenal insufficiency.

REFERENCES
1   Sweeney AT, Malabanan AO, Blake MA *et al.* Megacolon as the presenting feature in pheochromocytoma. *J Clin Endocrinol Metab.* 2000; **85**(11): 3968–72.

2 Valenzuela GA, Smalley WE, Schain DC *et al.* Reversibility of gastric dysmotility in cortisol deficiency. *Am J Gastroenterol.* 1987; **82**(10): 1066–8.

3 Gunsar F, Yilmaz S, Bor S *et al.* Effect of hypo- and hyperthyroidism on gastric myoelectrical activity. *Dig Dis Sci.* 2003; **48**(4): 706–12.

CHAPTER 15

Gastrointestinal haemorrhage

PATHOPHYSIOLOGY AND AETIOLOGY

Bleeding from the gastrointestinal (GI) tract is a common reason for acute medical admission. It may present with the vomiting of fresh blood, or of altered blood that has the appearance of coffee grounds. Alternatively, the passage per rectum of fresh blood or black altered blood (melaena) may be noted. More insidious bleeding may cause iron-deficiency anaemia with no other symptoms. Gastrointestinal bleeding may arise from conditions that are localised to one part of the gut, or from more generalised conditions that can potentially affect the whole GI tract. The main mechanisms responsible for gastrointestinal bleeding are mechanical, chemical or radiation injury, neoplasia, infection, inflammation, vascular disorders and other structural disorders.

Table 15.1 lists the causes of gastrointestinal haemorrhage, with common causes highlighted in bold type.

EMERGENCY MANAGEMENT

➤ Assess the airway:
  – Use suction to clear blood or vomitus from the mouth, and place the patient in the left lateral position to prevent aspiration.
  – Oropharyngeal or nasopharyngeal airway adjuncts may be required if consciousness is impaired. In some cases tracheal intubation may be required.
➤ Breathing:
  – Correct hypoxia with high-flow oxygen.
  – Provide antibiotics for aspiration pneumonia if this is detected.
➤ Circulation:
  – Obtain reliable intravenous access by means of two large-bore peripheral cannulae, and send blood for urgent cross-matching.
  – If the patient is hypovolaemic, provide fluid resuscitation with packed red cells. In moderate cases, colloid and normal saline may be used for resuscitation while awaiting delivery of packed red cells from the blood bank. However, in severe cases the emergency supply of O-negative packed red cells should be utilised.
➤ Control the bleeding:
  – Correct any coagulopathy and reverse anticoagulation if possible; in complex cases such as GI bleeding in a patient with a prosthetic mitral valve, the appropriate specialists should be consulted for advice.
  – IV terlipressin should be given in cases of variceal haemorrhage; IV proton pump inhibitor (e.g. esomeprazole) should be strongly considered in acute severe upper GI bleeding.
  – Sengstaken–Blakemore tube insertion may be required to control bleeding from oesophageal varices pending definitive treatment.
  – Endoscopic treatment includes the banding or injection of oesophageal varices and the injection of peptic ulcers with sclerosing agents.
  – Surgical treatment may be required (e.g. to oversew a bleeding peptic ulcer).
  – Selective arteriography with embolisation of the bleeding vessel or intra-arterial vasopressin injection is a further treatment option for intractable haemorrhage.

HISTORY

➤ Presenting complaint:
  – Haematemesis, coffee-ground vomiting and melaena suggest upper GI bleeding.
  – Fresh rectal bleeding suggests a lower GI source, or very brisk upper GI bleeding.
  – Anaemia with no other symptoms may occur with more insidious bleeding.
➤ Duration of symptoms.
➤ Associated symptoms:
  – Syncope, confusion, oliguria and thirst suggest hypovolaemia.
  – Pallor, shortness of breath and fatigue are symptoms of anaemia.
  – Abdominal pain may occur with inflammatory bowel disease, peptic ulcer disease, gastroenteritis and bowel ischaemia.
➤ Drug history. Note in particular any use of NSAIDs, warfarin or antiplatelet agents.

Table 15.1 Causes of gastrointestinal haemorrhage

Anatomically localised disorders

Oesophageal, gastric and duodenal	*Small bowel*	*Large bowel*
Mucosal damage ▲ Mallory-Weiss tear ▲ Oesophagitis ▲ Gastritis ▲ Peptic ulcer disease ▲ Gastric volvulus ▲ Eosinophilic gastroenteritis Vascular ▲ Oesophageal varices ▲ Gastric varices ▲ Gastric antral vascular ectasia ▲ Dieulafoy's lesion ▲ Portal hypertensive gastropathy Neoplasia ▲ Gastric cancer ▲ Lymphoma ▲ Miscellaneous	Crohn's disease Coeliac disease Acute mesenteric ischaemia Structural disorders ▲ Meckel's diverticulum ▲ Intussusception ▲ Diverticulosis ▲ Cronkhite-Canada syndrome ▲ Idiopathic ulcerative enteritis ▲ Haemobilia ▲ Haemosuccus pancreaticus ▲ Cholecystoduodenal fistula Neoplasia ▲ Benign tumours ▲ Adenocarcinoma ▲ Lymphoma ▲ Miscellaneous	Structural disorders ▲ Diverticulosis ▲ Caecal ulcer ▲ Solitary rectal ulcer syndrome ▲ Stercoral ulcer ▲ Pneumatosis intestinalis ▲ Colitis cystica profunda Inflammation ▲ Ulcerative colitis ▲ Crohn's disease ▲ Neutropenic colitis ▲ Drug-induced colitis Vascular disorders ▲ Haemorrhoids ▲ Angiodysplasia ▲ Ischaemic colitis ▲ Colonic varices Neoplasia ▲ Colorectal cancer ▲ Colorectal adenoma ▲ Anal cancer ▲ Miscellaneous Infection ▲ Enteroinvasive or enterohaemorrhagic *E. coli* ▲ *Shigella* ▲ *Campylobacter* ▲ Pseudomembranous colitis ▲ Amoebic dysentery ▲ Miscellaneous

Generalised disorders

Vascular disorders	*Infection*	*Extrinsic insults*
Vascular malformations ▲ Hereditary haemorrhagic telangiectasia ▲ Angiodysplasia ▲ Varices ▲ Dieulafoy's lesion ▲ Haemangioma ▲ BRBNS ▲ Aortoenteric fistula Small vessel vasculopathy ▲ Henoch-Schönlein purpura ▲ Polyarteritis nodosa ▲ Microscopic polyangiitis ▲ Churg-Strauss syndrome ▲ Behçet's disease ▲ Cryoglobulinaemia ▲ Systemic lupus erythematosus ▲ Cholesterol embolism ▲ Degos' disease ▲ Miscellaneous Connective tissue disease ▲ Amyloidosis ▲ Ehlers-Danlos syndrome ▲ Pseudoxanthoma elasticum ▲ Menke's disease	Viral haemorrhagic fever Bacterial infection ▲ Tuberculosis ▲ Leptospirosis ▲ Typhoid fever ▲ Tularaemia ▲ Brucellosis ▲ Anthrax ▲ Whipple's disease Fungal infection ▲ Histoplasmosis ▲ Mucormycosis ▲ Paracoccidioidomycosis ▲ Candidiasis ▲ Penicilliosis Helminth infection ▲ Strongyloidiasis ▲ Hookworm ▲ Ascariasis ▲ Anisakiasis ▲ Trichuriasis ▲ Schistosomiasis ▲ Angiostrongyliasis Malaria	Drugs ▲ Warfarin ▲ NSAIDs ▲ Antiplatelet agents Toxins ▲ Iron salts ▲ Chromium salts ▲ Heavy metals ▲ Chemotherapy Miscellaneous ▲ Graft-versus-host disease ▲ Radiation enteritis ▲ Foreign body

➤ Alcohol history. Excessive alcohol intake predisposes to peptic ulcer disease, as well as to liver cirrhosis which may be complicated by oesophageal varices.
➤ Foreign travel. Bacterial or amoebic dysentery may occur in travellers returning from the tropics.

EXAMINATION
➤ Ensure that the airway is not compromised by vomitus or blood.
➤ Breathing:
 – Check oxygen saturations and respiratory rate.
 – Auscultate the chest for signs of aspiration pneumonia.
➤ Circulation:
 – Check for signs of hypovolaemia. These include tachycardia, tachypnoea, hypotension or postural hypotension, oliguria, confusion, weak thready pulse, cool peripheries, prolonged capillary refill time, reduced skin turgor, dry mucous membranes and low JVP.
➤ General examination:
 – Fever suggests an infective or inflammatory cause of bleeding, such as infective colitis or inflammatory bowel disease. Aspiration pneumonia is a further possible cause of fever.
 – Signs of chronic liver disease may be seen in cases of variceal bleeding. These include jaundice, clubbing, palmar erythema, hepatic flap, spider naevi and gynaecomastia.
 – Supraclavicular lymphadenopathy may occur in association with gastrointestinal malignancy.
 – Purpuric skin rash suggests systemic vasculitis or a bleeding disorder.
 – Widespread telangiectasia occurs with hereditary haemorrhagic telangiectasia.
 – Perioral pigmentation occurs with Peutz–Jeghers syndrome, which causes multiple small bowel polyps.
➤ Abdominal examination:
 – Severe tenderness or peritonism suggests a perforated viscus or bowel ischaemia.
 – A palpable abdominal mass may represent GI malignancy.
 – Splenomegaly occurs with liver cirrhosis, suggesting the possibility of oesophageal varices.
 – Abdominal aortic aneurysm may be palpable. Aortoenteric fistula is a rare but often fatal cause of GI bleeding.
 – Rectal examination may reveal melaena, fresh blood or a rectal tumour.

INVESTIGATIONS
➤ Blood tests:
 – FBC
 – clotting screen
 – U&Es – urea rises disproportionately in relation to creatinine with upper gastrointestinal haemorrhage, due to the absorbed protein load
 – LFTs may be deranged with chronic liver disease
 – CRP levels rise with infection or inflammation
 – lactate levels rise with acute mesenteric ischaemia or ischaemic colitis
 – tissue transglutaminase, anti-endomysial antibodies and anti-gliadin antibodies are found in coeliac disease.
➤ Stool culture and microscopy for ova and parasites is performed in cases of infective diarrhoea.
➤ CXR may reveal aspiration pneumonia.
➤ Gastrointestinal tract imaging with or without biopsy:
 – OGD is performed in cases of upper GI bleeding for both diagnostic and therapeutic purposes.
 – Flexible sigmoidoscopy is performed in cases of acute lower GI bleeding.
 – Colonoscopy or CT colonography allows visualisation of the entire colon. This is essential in the investigation of occult anaemia in order to detect right-sided colonic cancers.
 – Capsule enteroscopy is used to image the small bowel if no cause of bleeding is demonstrated during the initial investigations.
 – Angiography or CT angiography may be used to localise the feeding vessel to a bleeding point in the gut. The culprit vessel may then be occluded by embolisation or intra-arterial vasopressin injection.

CHAPTER 16

Dysphagia

PATHOPHYSIOLOGY AND AETIOLOGY

The causes of dysphagia (difficulty in swallowing) may be classified into neuromuscular and obstructive categories. Disruption of the neuromuscular control of swallowing may occur at the level of the central nervous system, the peripheral nerves or the pharyngeal and oesophageal muscles. Mechanical obstruction may be either intrinsic or extrinsic to the pharynx and oesophagus.

The causes of dysphagia are listed in Table 16.1, with common causes highlighted in bold type.

EMERGENCY MANAGEMENT

➤ Assess the airway (see Chapter 3). Epiglottitis is an uncommon but serious condition that may cause absolute dysphagia with compromise of the airway. Anaphylaxis and angioedema may also result in airway oedema and obstruction. Urgent anaesthetic review is mandatory if the patency of the airway is in doubt.

➤ Patients with neuromuscular dysphagia may be at risk of aspiration if they are allowed unrestricted oral intake. Therefore they should not eat or drink until the safety of the swallow has been formally assessed.

HISTORY

➤ Duration and pattern of symptoms.

➤ Speed of onset. Sudden onset is characteristic of foreign body impaction, whereas a slowly progressive course is more typical of malignant obstruction.

➤ Dysphagia to liquids or both liquids and solids is characteristic of neuromuscular disease, whereas mechanical obstruction usually causes dysphagia to solids only, unless the occlusion is complete or nearly so.

➤ History of foreign body ingestion or impaction of a food bolus.

➤ Associated symptoms:
  – Stridor or dyspnoea may indicate incipient airway obstruction.
  – Sore throat suggests pharyngeal infection, inflammation or neoplasia.
  – Substernal pain following swallowing occurs with oesophageal infection, inflammation or neoplasia.
  – Aspiration occurs with neuromuscular dysfunction or tracheo-oesophageal fistula.
  – Weakness, abnormal movement or altered sensation suggests a neuromuscular cause of dysphagia.

EXAMINATION

➤ General examination.
  – Fever suggests pharyngeal or oesophageal infection.
  – Cachexia is usually associated with malignant obstruction, but may occur with any form of chronic severe dysphagia.
  – Cervical lymphadenopathy may occur with oesophageal or gastric malignancy.
  – A palpable neck mass may represent goitre, thyroid or parathyroid tumour, or thyroglossal cyst.
  – Fixed, engorged neck veins suggest a mediastinal mass with SVC obstruction.
  – Signs of systemic sclerosis include tight skin, microstomia, nailfold telangiectasia, calcinosis and Raynaud's phenomenon.
  – Skin rash may occur with SLE, dermatomyositis or other connective tissue disorders.

➤ Examination of the mouth and pharynx should not be performed without anaesthetic support and full resuscitation facilities if airway compromise is a possibility, as it may precipitate complete airway occlusion. This is particularly applicable to patients with infective or inflammatory disease of the oropharynx, such as epiglottitis, angioedema or anaphylaxis.

➤ Neurological examination:
  – Weakness or muscle wasting suggests a myopathy or neuromuscular junction disorder.
  – Ptosis is most commonly associated with myasthenia gravis, but may occur with other myopathies and disorders of the neuromuscular junction.
  – Cranial nerves. A lower motor neuron lesion of cranial nerves IX, X, XI and XII (bulbar palsy) is caused by damage to the cranial nerves or nerve roots, whereas an upper motor neuron lesion (pseudobulbar palsy) is caused by damage to the corticobulbar tract. Bulbar palsy is characterised by

Table 16.1 Causes of dysphagia

Neuromuscular dysfunction

Central nervous system

Vascular
- ➤ Brainstem infarction
- ➤ Brainstem haemorrhage
- ➤ Vertebrobasilar insufficiency

Space-occupying lesion
- ➤ Brainstem tumour
- ➤ Brainstem abscess

Demyelination
- ➤ Multiple sclerosis
- ➤ ADEM
- ➤ CPM
- ➤ PML

Degenerative
- ➤ Parkinson's disease
- ➤ Progressive supranuclear palsy
- ➤ Multiple system atrophy
- ➤ Corticobasal degeneration
- ➤ Miscellaneous

Inherited/congenital
- ➤ Huntington's disease
- ➤ Wilson's disease
- ➤ Neuroferritinopathy
- ➤ Leukodystrophies
- ➤ Spinocerebellar ataxias
- ➤ Friedrich's ataxia
- ➤ Chiari malformation
- ➤ Miscellaneous

Miscellaneous
- ➤ Viral encephalitis
- ➤ CNS vasculitis
- ➤ Paraneoplastic brainstem encephalitis
- ➤ Hashimoto's encephalopathy
- ➤ Stiff person syndrome
- ➤ Neuroleptic malignant syndrome
- ➤ Status dystonicus
- ➤ Strychnine toxicity
- ➤ Tetanus

Peripheral nerve

Motor neuron disease

Diabetes mellitus

Compression or damage
- ➤ Thyroid surgery
- ➤ Lung cancer
- ➤ Glomus tumour
- ➤ Syringobulbia
- ➤ Radiation
- ➤ Miscellaneous

Infection
- ➤ Poliomyelitis
- ➤ Herpes zoster
- ➤ Diphtheria
- ➤ Lyme disease
- ➤ Leprosy
- ➤ Neurosyphilis
- ➤ Tuberculous meningitis
- ➤ Miscellaneous

Inflammation
- ➤ Guillain–Barré syndrome
- ➤ CIDP
- ➤ Sarcoidosis
- ➤ Vasculitis
- ➤ Connective tissue disease
- ➤ Paraneoplastic neuropathy
- ➤ CANOMAD syndrome
- ➤ Cranial pachymeningitis

Charcot–Marie–Tooth disease

Acute intermittent porphyria

Lead poisoning

Muscle

Oesophageal dysmotility
- ➤ Achalasia
- ➤ Spastic motility disorders
- ➤ Chagas' disease
- ➤ Trichinosis
- ➤ Acute intravascular haemolysis[1]

Inflammation
- ➤ Systemic sclerosis
- ➤ Systemic lupus erythematosus
- ➤ Mixed connective tissue disease
- ➤ Sjögren's syndrome
- ➤ Polymyositis
- ➤ Dermatomyositis
- ➤ Inclusion body myositis

Toxic, endocrine or metabolic
- ➤ Alcoholic myopathy
- ➤ Diabetes mellitus
- ➤ Hypo/hyperthyroidism
- ➤ Hypocalcaemia
- ➤ Hypomagnesaemia
- ➤ Amyloidosis
- ➤ Miscellaneous

Inherited myopathies
- ➤ Myotonic dystrophy
- ➤ Muscular dystrophy
- ➤ Glycogen storage diseases
- ➤ Mitochondrial myopathies
- ➤ Miscellaneous

Neuromuscular junction disorders
- ➤ Myasthenia gravis
- ➤ LEMS
- ➤ Botulism
- ➤ Marine neurotoxins
- ➤ Tick paralysis
- ➤ Envenomation
- ➤ Organophosphates
- ➤ Congenital myasthenic syndromes

Obstruction

Intrinsic

Foreign body

Oesophagitis
- ➤ GORD
- ➤ Infection
- ➤ Medication
- ➤ Radiation
- ➤ Caustic ingestion
- ➤ Eosinophilic oesophagitis
- ➤ Miscellaneous

Neoplasia
- ➤ Oesophageal
- ➤ Pharyngeal
- ➤ Gastric

Structural abnormalities
- ➤ Oesophageal diverticula
- ➤ Pharyngeal pouch
- ➤ Rings or webs
- ➤ Tracheo-oesophageal fistula
- ➤ Cricoarytenoid arthritis
- ➤ Laryngopharyngeal reflux
- ➤ Gastric volvulus

Infection
- ➤ Quinsy
- ➤ Deep neck infections
- ➤ Epiglottitis
- ➤ Diphtheria
- ➤ Paracoccidioidomycosis

Hypersensitivity reactions
- ➤ Angioedema
- ➤ Anaphylaxis

Mucosal pathology
- ➤ Pemphigus
- ➤ Pemphigoid
- ➤ Epidermolysis bullosa
- ➤ Behçet's disease
- ➤ Toxic epidermal necrolysis

Extrinsic

Thyroid and parathyroid
- ➤ Goitre
- ➤ Thyroid cancer
- ➤ Thyroglossal cyst
- ➤ Parathyroid tumour

Mediastinal mass
- ➤ Thymoma
- ➤ Germ-cell tumour
- ➤ Neurogenic tumours
- ➤ Lymphoma
- ➤ Bronchogenic cyst
- ➤ Pericardial cyst
- ➤ Thoracic aortic aneurysm
- ➤ Miscellaneous

Miscellaneous
- ➤ Cervical spondylosis
- ➤ Sclerosing mediastinitis

nasal speech, tongue wasting and fasciculation, and an absent gag reflex. Pseudobulbar palsy is characterised by spastic dysarthria, a brisk gag reflex and jaw jerk, and emotional lability.
- Hemiparesis, hemisensory loss, dysphasia, dyspraxia, visual neglect or homonymous hemianopia suggest a cerebral lesion.
- Abnormal, uncoordinated or involuntary movement may occur with degenerative, demyelinating or inherited disorders of the central nervous system.

INVESTIGATIONS
The following core investigations are commonly required:
➤ Blood tests:
- FBC. Malignancy may cause anaemia of chronic disease.
- U&Es. Poor oral intake may result in dehydration and acute kidney injury.
- Glucose. Diabetes mellitus may cause peripheral and autonomic neuropathy, resulting in oesophageal dysmotility.
➤ Imaging:
- CXR should be performed if aspiration pneumonia is a possibility.
- OGD. Oropharyngeal, oesophageal and gastric lesions may be directly visualised and biopsied. Stenting of malignant strictures can also be performed.
- Barium swallow may reveal structural abnormalities of the oesophagus.

The following further investigations may be required:
➤ Blood tests:
- TFTs should be performed if a thyroid mass is present.
- Autoimmune screen. This should include ANA, anti-dsDNA (SLE), anti-centromere antibodies or anti-Scl-70 antibodies (systemic sclerosis), anti-RNP antibodies (mixed connective tissue disease) and anti-Jo-1 antibodies (polymyositis).
- VDRL and TPHA should be checked if neurosyphilis is suspected.
➤ Imaging:
- Lateral neck X-ray may reveal an enlarged epiglottis in epiglottitis.
- CT of the chest should be performed if a mediastinal mass is suspected.
- CT of the neck may reveal thyroid enlargement or other obstructing masses.
- Oesophageal manometry may be diagnostic of dysmotility disorders.
- Laryngoscopy allows direct visualisation of vocal cord movement. Abnormalities may be caused by lesions of the vagus nerve or recurrent laryngeal nerve.
- CT or MRI of the brain should be performed if a neurological cause of dysphagia is suspected. Haemorrhage, infarction, tumour or abscess may be diagnosed.
➤ The Tensilon test may be diagnostic of myasthenia gravis.

REFERENCE
1   Rother RP, Bell L, Hillmen P et al. The clinical sequelae of intravascular haemolysis and extracellular plasma haemoglobin. JAMA. 2005; 293: 1653–62.

CHAPTER 17

Diarrhoea

PATHOPHYSIOLOGY AND AETIOLOGY

Diarrhoea may be defined as the abnormal passage of loose or liquid stools more than three times daily and/or a volume of stool greater than 200 g/day.[1]

The mechanisms of diarrhoea may be summarised as follows:

1 **Increased secretion of fluid into the colon.** This is most often due to infection, inflammation or tumour. Neuroendocrine causes such as carcinoid syndrome are less common.

2 **Colonic mucosal damage.** This is usually due to infection or inflammation. It results in decreased ability of the colon to absorb fluid.

3 **Colonic hypermotility.** This may be induced by infection or neuroendocrine conditions such as hyperthyroidism. The reduced transit time of stool through the large bowel results in less opportunity for colonic fluid absorption.

4 **Osmotic diarrhoea.** The presentation of hyperosmolar small bowel contents to the colon (e.g. due to malabsorption) results in water retention within the bowel due to the osmotic force exerted by the extra solutes.

The causes of diarrhoea are listed in Table 17.1, with common causes highlighted in bold type.

EMERGENCY MANAGEMENT

➤ Check for signs of hypovolaemia. These include tachycardia, tachypnoea, hypotension or postural hypotension, oliguria, confusion, weak thready pulse, cool peripheries, prolonged capillary refill time, reduced skin turgor, dry mucous membranes and low JVP. Provide fluid resuscitation with normal saline with or without potassium as appropriate.

➤ Acute flares of inflammatory bowel disease require treatment with systemic steroids with or without steroid enemas. Early surgical review should be sought, as severe cases that do not respond to medical management may require colectomy.

➤ Pseudomembranous colitis is a severe form of *Clostridium difficile* infection. It is treated with oral metronidazole or vancomycin according to local guidelines. Early surgical review should be sought, as some cases progress to toxic megacolon with possible bowel perforation.

HISTORY

➤ Details of the diarrhoea:
  – Duration of symptoms.
  – Diurnal variation. Opening the bowels at night suggests organic pathology.
  – Appearance of the stool. The presence of blood or mucus suggests infective, inflammatory or neoplastic pathology of the colon. Offensive stool that is difficult to flush suggests malabsorption with steatorrhoea. Pale stool occurs with obstructive jaundice. Silver stool classically occurs with chronic pancreatitis.

➤ Associated symptoms:
  – Fever suggests infection or inflammation.
  – Abdominal pain may occur with a variety of infectious, inflammatory or ischaemic bowel conditions.
  – Vomiting with diarrhoea is commonly caused by viral gastroenteritis.
  – Tenesmus may occur with rectal carcinoma or colonic villous adenoma.
  – Drug history. Take particular note of recent courses of antibiotics, as these predispose to antibiotic-associated diarrhoea and *Clostridium difficile* infection.
  – Dietary history. Enquire about any recent dietary indiscretions, such as eating undercooked meat. Ask whether the patient's friends or relatives who have eaten the same food have also fallen ill.
  – Foreign travel. A number of pathogens, such as *Giardia lamblia*, can cause diarrhoea in the returning traveller.
  – Sexual history. Proctitis, for instance due to rectal gonorrhoea, may cause the frequent passage of mucoid stool.

EXAMINATION

General examination:
  – Check for signs of hypovolaemia.

Table 17.1 Causes of diarrhoea

Gastrointestinal disease	*Malabsorption*	*Systemic disease*

Gastrointestinal disease

Colonic infection

Viral infection
- ➤ Viral gastroenteritis
- ➤ CMV colitis
- ➤ HSV colitis

Bacterial infection
- ➤ *Salmonella*
- ➤ *Shigella*
- ➤ *Campylobacter*
- ➤ *E. coli*
- ➤ Pseudomembranous colitis
- ➤ *Listeria monocytogenes*
- ➤ Yersiniosis
- ➤ Typhoid fever
- ➤ Brucellosis
- ➤ Tularaemia
- ➤ Anthrax
- ➤ Tuberculosis
- ➤ Atypical mycobacteria
- ➤ Cholera
- ➤ Non-cholera vibrios
- ➤ *Aeromonas*
- ➤ *Plesiomonas*
- ➤ Rectal gonorrhoea
- ➤ Rectal primary syphilis
- ➤ Lymphogranuloma venereum

Protozoan infection
- ➤ Amoebic colitis
- ➤ Cryptosporidiosis
- ➤ Isosporiasis
- ➤ Microsporidiosis
- ➤ Cyclosporiasis
- ➤ Balantidiasis
- ➤ Sarcocystosis
- ➤ *Blastocystis hominis*
- ➤ Visceral leishmaniasis

Miscellaneous colonic disease

Neoplasia
- ➤ Colorectal carcinoma
- ➤ Villous colonic adenoma

Local colonic inflammation
- ➤ Ulcerative colitis
- ➤ Crohn's disease
- ➤ Diverticulitis
- ➤ Acute appendicitis
- ➤ Ischaemic colitis
- ➤ Lymphocytic colitis
- ➤ Collagenous colitis
- ➤ Radiation colitis
- ➤ Neutropenic colitis
- ➤ Chemotherapy
- ➤ Drug-induced colitis
- ➤ Colonic malakoplakia
- ➤ Endometriosis

Systemic inflammation with colonic involvement
- ➤ Systemic lupus erythematosus
- ➤ Churg–Strauss syndrome
- ➤ Microscopic polyangiitis
- ➤ Polyarteritis nodosa
- ➤ Behçet's disease
- ➤ Mastocytosis
- ➤ Hypereosinophilic syndrome
- ➤ Graft-versus-host disease
- ➤ HIDS
- ➤ Degos' disease
- ➤ Miscellaneous

Structural abnormalities
- ➤ Pneumatosis intestinalis
- ➤ Colitis cystica profunda

Malabsorption

Pancreatic disease
- ➤ Chronic pancreatitis
- ➤ Pancreatic carcinoma
- ➤ Cystic fibrosis
- ➤ Miscellaneous

Biliary disease
- ➤ Bile salt malabsorption
- ➤ Biliary obstruction
- ➤ Biliary atresia
- ➤ Liver cirrhosis

Gastric disease
- ➤ Gastric carcinoma
- ➤ Atrophic gastritis
- ➤ Post-gastrectomy syndrome

- ➤ Acquired small bowel disease
- ➤ Coeliac disease
- ➤ Small bowel bacterial overgrowth
- ➤ Giardiasis
- ➤ Short bowel syndrome
- ➤ Jejunoileal bypass
- ➤ Mesenteric ischaemia
- ➤ Gastrointestinal lymphoma
- ➤ Cronkhite–Canada syndrome
- ➤ Alpha heavy-chain disease
- ➤ Amyloidosis
- ➤ Whipple's disease
- ➤ Tropical sprue
- ➤ Helminth infection
- ➤ Eosinophilic enteritis
- ➤ Autoimmune enteropathy
- ➤ Collagenous sprue
- ➤ Chemotherapy
- ➤ Drug-induced malabsorption
- ➤ Radiation enteritis

Systemic disease

Autonomic neuropathy

Endocrine and metabolic
- ➤ **Hyperthyroidism**
- ➤ **Diabetes mellitus**
- ➤ Carcinoid syndrome
- ➤ Glucagonoma
- ➤ Somatostinoma
- ➤ VIPoma
- ➤ Gastrinoma
- ➤ Hypoparathyroidism
- ➤ Medullary thyroid carcinoma
- ➤ Adrenal insufficiency
- ➤ Congenital chloridorrhoea
- ➤ Pellagra

Drugs
- ➤ **Proton pump inhibitors**
- ➤ **Antibiotics**
- ➤ **Laxatives**
- ➤ Enteral feeding
- ➤ Miscellaneous

Food-borne bacterial toxins
- ➤ *Staphylococcus aureus*
- ➤ *Bacillus cereus*
- ➤ *Clostridium perfringens*
- ➤ *Clostridium botulinum*

Miscellaneous toxins
- ➤ Arsenic
- ➤ Carbon monoxide
- ➤ Organophosphates
- ➤ Toxic plants or seafood
- ➤ Beer excess
- ➤ Miscellaneous

Table 17.1 Causes of diarrhoea – *continued*

Gastrointestinal disease

Colonic infection	*Miscellaneous colonic disease*	*Osmotic diarrhoea*	*Systemic disease*
Fungal infection	Functional	➤ Idiopathic ulcerative enteritis	Toxic shock syndrome
➤ Paracoccidioidomycosis	➤ Irritable bowel syndrome	➤ HIV enteropathy	Systemic infection
➤ Histoplasmosis	➤ Functional diarrhoea	➤ Intestinal lymphangiectasia	
➤ Mucormycosis	➤ Overflow diarrhoea	➤ Protein-losing enteropathy	
➤ Candidiasis			
➤ Penicilliosis		Inherited small bowel disease	
		➤ Disaccharidase deficiency	
Trichuriasis		➤ Glucose-galactose malabsorption	
		➤ Fructose malabsorption	
		➤ IgA deficiency	
		➤ Abetalipoproteinaemia	
		➤ Hypoapobetalipoproteinaemia	
		➤ Lysinuric protein intolerance	
		➤ Hartnup disease	
		➤ Von Gierke's disease	
		➤ Fabry's disease	
		Drugs	
		➤ Lipase inhibitors	
		➤ α-glucosidase inhibitors	

- Anaemia occurs with malignancy, inflammatory bowel disease and coeliac disease.
- Supraclavicular lymphadenopathy may be present with gastrointestinal malignancy.
- Clubbing may be a feature of Crohn's disease.
➤ Abdominal examination:
  - Significant tenderness or signs of peritonism, such as guarding, rebound tenderness and absent bowel sounds, should prompt urgent surgical referral.
  - A palpable abdominal mass may represent gastrointestinal malignancy.
  - Rectal examination may reveal a rectal tumour, or faecal impaction that is causing overflow diarrhoea.

INVESTIGATIONS

The following core investigations are commonly required:
➤ Blood tests:
  - FBC. This may reveal anaemia. A raised WBC suggests infection.
  - U&Es. Severe diarrhoea may cause hypovolaemia and acute kidney injury.
  - CRP. Levels are raised with infection or inflammation.
  - LFTs. These may be abnormal with biliary disease.
  - TFTs. Hyperthyroidism is a cause of diarrhoea.
  - Glucose. Diabetes mellitus may cause autonomic neuropathy and thus diarrhoea.
➤ Microbiology:
  - Blood culture if the patient is febrile.
  - Stool culture and microscopy for ova and parasites.
  - Stool *Clostridium difficile* toxin test.

The following further investigations may be required:
➤ Serology and biochemistry:
  - HIV test. AIDS may present with a diarrhoeal illness (e.g. caused by cytomegalovirus colitis or cryptosporidiosis).
  - CMV serology and PCR.
  - Parasite serology.
  - Lactate levels are raised with ischaemic colitis and acute mesenteric ischaemia.
  - Vitamin B_{12}, folate, ferritin, albumin and calcium. Low levels suggest malabsorption.
  - Tissue transglutaminase, anti-endomysial antibodies and anti-gliadin antibodies are present in coeliac disease.
  - Faecal elastase. Activity of this enzyme is low in pancreatic exocrine insufficiency.
  - Stool and urine laxative screen.
  - Twenty-four-hour urine collection for 5 HIAA. Levels of this metabolite are raised with carcinoid syndrome.
  - Serum measurements of VIP, gastrin and glucagon may rarely be required to exclude endocrine causes of diarrhoea.
➤ Imaging:
  - Flexible sigmoidoscopy or colonoscopy allows the histological diagnosis to be obtained in cases of acute colitis. Diverticular disease may also be visualised.
  - OGD with duodenal biopsy may be diagnostic in cases of malabsorption.
  - CT of the abdomen may reveal gastrointestinal or pancreatic cancer.
➤ Specific tests of absorptive function are usually performed in a specialist setting.

REFERENCE
1   Thomas PD, Forbes A, Green J et al. Guidelines for the investigation of chronic diarrhoea, 2nd edition. *Gut*. 2003; **52 (Suppl. V):** v1–15.

CHAPTER 18

Constipation

PATHOPHYSIOLOGY AND AETIOLOGY

Constipation is the complaint of difficult defecation. It may be caused by the following mechanisms:

1   mechanical bowel obstruction
2   impaired neurological control of bowel motility
3   toxic, endocrine or metabolic derangements resulting in reduced bowel motility
4   lifestyle factors or functional disorders.

The causes of constipation are listed in Table 18.1, with common causes highlighted in bold type.

EMERGENCY MANAGEMENT

➤   Absolute constipation, which is the failure to pass faeces or flatus, is indicative of bowel obstruction, and urgent surgical referral is mandatory.

➤   Change in bowel habit in association with low back pain may be due to cauda equina syndrome, which is a neurosurgical emergency. If this condition is suspected, an urgent MRI of the spine should be performed and a neurosurgical review arranged.

Table 18.1 Causes of constipation

Mechanical	Toxic, endocrine and metabolic	Neurological	Lifestyle factors and functional disorders
Anorectal conditions	Peritonitis	Cerebral	Lifestyle factors
➤ **Faecal impaction**		➤ **Stroke**	➤ **Low-fibre diet**
➤ **Anal fissure**	Drugs and toxins	➤ **Parkinson's disease**	➤ **Immobility**
➤ Anorectal abscess	➤ **Opiates**		➤ **Pregnancy**
➤ Anal carcinoma	➤ **Anticholinergics**	Spinal	
➤ Anal stricture	➤ Lead	➤ **Multiple sclerosis**	Functional
➤ Lichen sclerosus	➤ Miscellaneous	➤ **Tumour**	➤ **Depression**
➤ Rectal prolapse		➤ Trauma	➤ **Irritable bowel**
➤ Solitary rectal ulcer	Endocrine/metabolic	➤ Miscellaneous	**syndrome**
➤ Lymphogranuloma	➤ **Hypothyroidism**		➤ Slow-transit constipation
venereum	➤ **Diabetes mellitus**	Peripheral nerve	➤ Idiopathic megacolon
➤ Haemorrhoid	➤ Hypercalcaemia	➤ **Cauda equina**	➤ Anismus
	➤ Hypokalaemia	**syndrome**	
Bowel obstruction	➤ Acute porphyria	➤ Sacral plexus damage	
➤ **Tumour**	➤ Phaeochromocytoma		
➤ **Adhesions**	➤ Adrenal insufficiency	Enteric nervous system	
➤ Stricture	➤ Ovarian carcinoid[1]	➤ **Ileus**	
➤ Incarcerated hernia	➤ Anorexia nervosa	➤ Ogilvie's syndrome	
➤ **Diverticulosis**	➤ Beriberi	➤ Chronic intestinal	
➤ Acute appendicitis		pseudo-obstruction	
➤ Volvulus		➤ Hirschsprung's disease	
➤ Intussusception		➤ Systemic sclerosis	
➤ Gallstone ileus		➤ Mixed connective tissue	
➤ Endometriosis		disease	
➤ Sclerosing peritonitis		➤ Amyloidosis	
➤ Retroperitoneal fibrosis		➤ Botulism	
➤ Typhoid fever		➤ Chagas' disease	
➤ Helminth infection		➤ Autonomic neuropathy	
		➤ Myotonic dystrophy	
Extrinsic compression		➤ Familial visceral	
➤ Ovarian tumour		myopathy	
➤ Uterine fibroid		➤ Miscellaneous	
➤ Uterine prolapse			
➤ Miscellaneous			

HISTORY
➤ Note the duration of symptoms and the time since the bowels were last open.
➤ Enquire about the current frequency of defecation as compared with the usual frequency.
➤ Ask whether flatus is being passed. The absence of flatus implies mechanical bowel obstruction.
➤ Associated symptoms:
  – Painful defecation is associated with a number of anorectal conditions, particularly anal fissures.
  – Vomiting, abdominal distension and colicky abdominal pain suggest mechanical bowel obstruction.
  – Back pain, lower limb weakness or numbness, perineal numbness and urinary disturbances such as incontinence or retention suggest cauda equina syndrome.
➤ Drug history. Particular note should be made of the use of opiates.
➤ Dietary history. A low-fibre diet predisposes to constipation.

EXAMINATION
➤ Abdominal examination:
  – A palpable mass may represent a faecally loaded colon or an obstructing malignancy. Faeces are indentable by the examining finger, whereas tumours are not.
  – Signs of peritonism, such as guarding, rigidity, rebound tenderness and percussion tenderness, suggest a perforated viscus, and urgent surgical referral is mandatory.
  – Auscultate the bowel sounds. Absent bowel sounds suggest reduced colonic motility (e.g. due to peritonitis or paralytic ileus). High-pitched active bowel sounds imply mechanical obstruction.
  – Examine the hernial orifices carefully. An incarcerated inguinal or femoral hernia is a common cause of small bowel obstruction.
  – Perform a rectal examination. This may reveal faecal impaction, rectal carcinoma or a variety of other anorectal conditions. Check for anal sphincter tone and perianal sensation. Loss of tone or sensation may herald cauda equina syndrome.
➤ Neurological examination:
  – Lower spinal cord pathology may cause spastic paraparesis or loss of lower limb sensation.
  – Cauda equina syndrome is associated with flaccid lower limb weakness and loss of lower limb sensation.

INVESTIGATIONS
The following core investigations are commonly required:
➤ Blood tests:
  – FBC. Anaemia may occur with colorectal cancer.
  – U&Es and calcium. Hypokalaemia and hypercalcaemia are causes of constipation.
  – CRP. Levels are raised with infection or inflammation.
  – TFTs. Hypothyroidism is a cause of constipation.
  – Glucose. Diabetes mellitus may cause autonomic neuropathy and consequently constipation.
➤ Imaging:
  – Plain abdominal X-ray should be performed if bowel obstruction is suspected. Dilated bowel loops or a volvulus may be visualised.
  – An erect CXR may reveal subdiaphragmatic air, which is a feature of bowel perforation.

The following further investigations may be required:
➤ Imaging:
  – CT of the abdomen provides further diagnostic information in cases of bowel obstruction or peritonitis, and helps to guide subsequent surgery.
  – Flexible sigmoidoscopy or colonoscopy may reveal tumours or diverticulosis.
  – MRI of the spine should be performed urgently if spinal cord pathology or cauda equina syndrome is suspected.
➤ Stool microscopy for ova and parasites may be required if there has been previous travel to an area where parasitic infection is endemic.

REFERENCE
1   Motoyama T, Kafayama Y, Watanabe H *et al.* Functioning ovarian carcinoids induce severe constipation. *Cancer.* 1992; **70**: 513–18.

CHAPTER 19

Abdominal swelling

PATHOPHYSIOLOGY AND AETIOLOGY

Generalised swelling of the abdomen is most often caused by ascites, bowel dilatation, pregnancy or obesity. Bladder distension, massive organomegaly and large intra-abdominal cysts or tumours may also result in noticeable abdominal distension. The causes of bowel obstruction are covered in Chapters 13 and 14.

Ascites may be defined as an abnormal accumulation of fluid within the abdominal cavity. The causes of ascites may be divided into three broad categories:

1 portal hypertension
2 peritoneal disease
3 miscellaneous causes.

The serum ascites albumin gradient (SAAG), which is the difference between the serum and ascitic fluid albumin concentrations, is useful in the diagnosis of ascites.[1]

Portal hypertension causes ascites with an SAAG of > 11 g/l, due to increased gastrointestinal tract capillary bed pressure, which forces fluid out of the circulation and into the peritoneal cavity. Other factors that may contribute in the case of liver cirrhosis include reduced plasma oncotic pressure due to hypoalbuminaemia, and sodium and water retention due to vasodilatation and renin–angiotensin system activation. Peritoneal disease, due to infection, inflammation or malignancy, tends to produce ascites with an SAAG of < 11g/L. The miscellaneous category is a diverse group of conditions, so the SAAG may be either low or high. The causes of ascites are listed in Table 19.1, with common causes highlighted in bold type.

EMERGENCY MANAGEMENT

Spontaneous bacterial peritonitis must be ruled in or out in any acutely unwell patient with ascites. The diagnosis should be made on the basis of an ascitic fluid neutrophil count of > 250 cells/μl, positive ascitic fluid culture or clinical suspicion. Treatment is with a broad-spectrum antibiotic that provides Gram-negative cover. Third-generation cephalosporins such as cefotaxime are most commonly used.[1]

HISTORY

➤ Time course of symptoms.
➤ Associated symptoms:
 – Abdominal pain and fever occur with spontaneous bacterial peritonitis.
 – Jaundice suggests decompensated liver cirrhosis or fulminant hepatic failure.
 – Peripheral oedema, orthopnoea and paroxysmal nocturnal dyspnoea suggest a cardiac cause of ascites.
➤ Social history:
 – Alcohol intake.
 – Risk factors for hepatitis B and C infection include intravenous drug abuse, tattoos and high-risk sexual behaviour.

EXAMINATION

➤ General examination:
 – Signs of chronic liver disease include jaundice, spider naevi, gynaecomastia, palmar erythema, clubbing and hepatic flap.
 – Cachexia suggests malignancy.
 – Lymphadenopathy may occur with metastatic malignancy.
 – Peripheral oedema may be a feature of cardiac failure, liver cirrhosis or nephrotic syndrome.
➤ Abdominal examination:
 – Clinical signs of ascites include shifting dullness and fluid thrill.
 – Hepatomegaly may be caused by vascular congestion, whereas liver cirrhosis generally results in a shrunken liver.
 – Splenomegaly occurs with portal hypertension of any cause.
 – Bowel sounds are high-pitched and active with bowel obstruction, and reduced with paralytic ileus or peritonitis.
 – The hernial orifices should be examined carefully. An incarcerated hernia may cause small bowel obstruction.

Table 19.1 Causes of ascites[2]

Portal hypertension	*Peritoneal disease*	*Miscellaneous*
Liver cirrhosis	Neoplasia	Hypoalbuminaemia
➤ Alcoholic liver disease	➤ Mesothelioma	➤ Nephrotic syndrome
➤ Non-alcoholic steatohepatitis	➤ Pseudomyxoma peritonei	➤ Protein-losing enteropathy
➤ Hepatitis B or C	➤ Peritoneal metastases	➤ Malnutrition
➤ Autoimmune hepatitis	➤ Miscellaneous	
➤ Primary biliary cirrhosis		Miscellaneous
➤ Primary sclerosing cholangitis	Infection	➤ Ovarian cancer
➤ Biliary stricture	➤ Spontaneous bacterial peritonitis	➤ Benign ovarian tumours
➤ Caroli's disease	➤ Fitz–Hugh–Curtis syndrome	➤ Ovarian hyperstimulation syndrome
➤ Haemochromatosis	➤ Tuberculosis	➤ Acute pancreatitis
➤ Wilson's disease	➤ Fungal peritonitis	➤ Pancreatic pseudocyst
➤ α1-antitrypsin deficiency	➤ Strongyloidiasis	➤ Acute mesenteric ischaemia
➤ Miscellaneous	➤ Miscellaneous	➤ Hypothyroidism
		➤ Nephrogenic ascites
Acute hepatitis	Inflammation	➤ Peritoneal dialysis
➤ Viral	➤ Connective tissue disease	➤ Chylous ascites
➤ Alcoholic	➤ Vasculitis	➤ Haemorrhage
➤ Toxic	➤ Familial Mediterranean fever	➤ Endometriosis
➤ Miscellaneous	➤ Eosinophilic gastroenteritis	➤ Urine leak
	➤ Mastocytosis	➤ Bile leak
Cardiac disease	➤ AILD	
➤ Congestive cardiac failure	➤ Sarcoidosis	
➤ Cor pulmonale	➤ Degos' disease[4]	
➤ Constrictive pericarditis		
➤ Restrictive cardiomyopathy		
➤ Tricuspid regurgitation		
➤ Atrial myxoma		
➤ Primary pulmonary hypertension		
Vascular disease		
➤ Budd–Chiari syndrome		
➤ Veno-occlusive disease		
➤ Inferior vena cava obstruction		
➤ Portal vein obstruction		
➤ Hereditary haemorrhagic telangiectasia		
➤ Schistosomiasis		
Miscellaneous		
➤ Malignant liver infiltration		
➤ Nodular regenerative hyperplasia		
➤ Peliosis hepatis		
➤ Myelofibrosis		
➤ Amyloidosis[3]		

➤ Cardiovascular examination:
- Signs of cardiac failure include raised JVP, peripheral oedema and bi-basal inspiratory crackles.
- Constrictive pericarditis is associated with a raised JVP that rises further on inspiration (Kussmaul's sign). Auscultation may reveal a pericardial knock.
- Signs of tricuspid regurgitation include a raised JVP with giant V waves and a pansystolic murmur at the lower left sternal edge, which is loudest on inspiration.

INVESTIGATIONS
The following core investigations are commonly required:
➤ Blood tests:
- FBC. Anaemia occurs with malignancy, whereas a raised WBC suggests infection.
- CRP. Levels are raised with infection or inflammation.
- U&Es. Renal impairment may occur in association with cardiac or hepatic failure.
- LFTs.
- Raised INR and hypoalbuminaemia are features of hepatic failure.
➤ Urine dip. Heavy proteinuria suggests nephrotic syndrome.
➤ Pregnancy test.

➤ Ascitic fluid analysis:
  – albumin
  – amylase
  – MC&S
  – cytology.
➤ Imaging:
  – CXR may reveal pulmonary oedema, which suggests congestive cardiac failure.
  – Plain abdominal X-ray may show dilated large or small bowel.
  – USS or CT of the abdomen will confirm the presence of ascites or bowel obstruction, and may reveal the cause.

The following further investigations may be required:
➤ Blood tests:
  – Hepatitis A, B and C, EBV and CMV serology.
  – Liver autoimmune screen. Anti-smooth muscle and anti-liver/kidney microsomal antibodies are present in autoimmune hepatitis, whereas anti-mitochondrial antibodies occur in primary biliary cirrhosis.
  – Ferritin. Levels are raised in haemochromatosis.
  – Caeruloplasmin. Levels are low in Wilson's disease.
  – α1-antitrypsin. Levels are low in α1-AT deficiency.
  – Amylase. Activity of this enzyme is raised with acute pancreatitis.
  – Tumour markers. These include α-fetoprotein (hepatocellular carcinoma), CA 19-9 (ovarian cancer) and CEA (colorectal cancer).
➤ Imaging:
  – Doppler USS or MRI may be used to assess hepatic arterial or portal vein inflow and hepatic vein outflow.
  – Echocardiogram allows diagnosis of cardiac conditions that cause systemic venous hypertension and hepatic congestion.
➤ Liver biopsy may be required in cases of fulminant hepatic failure of unknown cause.

REFERENCES
1 Moore KP, Aithal GP. Guidelines on the management of ascites in cirrhosis. *Gut.* 2006; **55 (Suppl. 6):** vi1–12.
2 Arroyo V, Gines P, Ramon P *et al.* Pathogenesis, diagnosis and treatment of ascites in cirrhosis. In: Bircher J, Benhamou J, McIntyre N *et al. Oxford Textbook of Hepatology.* 2nd edn. Oxford: Oxford University Press; 1999. pp. 697–731.
3 Peters RA, Koukoulis G, Gimson A *et al.* Primary amyloidosis and severe intrahepatic cholestatic jaundice. *Gut.* 1994; **35**(9): 1322–5.
4 Caviness VS, Sagar P, Israel EJ *et al.* Case 38-2006: a 5-year-old boy with headache and abdominal pain. *NEJM.* 2006; **355:** 2575–84.

CHAPTER 20

Jaundice

PATHOPHYSIOLOGY AND AETIOLOGY

Bilirubin is a breakdown product of haem that is produced in the liver, spleen and other tissues. It is initially transported in a water-insoluble unconjugated form, bound to plasma proteins. In the liver, bilirubin is conjugated with glucuronic acid to form water-soluble conjugated bilirubin, which is then excreted in bile. Jaundice is a yellowish discoloration of the skin and sclerae caused by the accumulation of bilirubin in the bloodstream. The three main categories of jaundice are as follows:

1 **Unconjugated hyperbilirubinaemia.** This is caused either by increased haemolysis, saturating the mechanisms for the conjugation of bilirubin and resulting in an accumulation of unconjugated bilirubin in the bloodstream, or by defective hepatic conjugation of bilirubin with glucuronic acid.
2 **Intrinsic liver disease.** This results in a mixed conjugated and unconjugated hyperbilirubinaemia, due to a combination of impaired bilirubin conjugation and intrahepatic biliary tract obstruction.
3 **Extrahepatic cholestasis.** This results from extrahepatic biliary tract obstruction, leading to inability to excrete bilirubin in the bile, and thus an accumulation of conjugated bilirubin in the bloodstream.

The causes of jaundice are listed in Table 20.1, with common causes highlighted in bold type.

EMERGENCY MANAGEMENT

Fulminant hepatic failure is a medical emergency. Early discussion with the regional liver unit is mandatory, as liver transplantation may be required in severe cases. Intensive-care input is needed in many cases to provide support to the cardiovascular, respiratory and renal systems pending definitive treatment.

HISTORY

➤ Note the time course and pattern of symptoms. Fluctuating jaundice is characteristic of gallstone disease, whereas a gradual progressive course suggests malignancy.
➤ Associated symptoms:
  - Pale stools and dark urine occur with extrahepatic cholestasis.
  - Red or brown urine may be caused by any condition that results in intravascular haemolysis and thus haemoglobinuria (e.g. paroxysmal nocturnal haemoglobinuria and malaria).
  - Fever and rigors suggest sepsis.
  - Abdominal pain occurs in a variety of conditions (e.g. acute cholangitis and alcoholic hepatitis).
  - Weight loss suggests malignancy.
  - Pruritus may occur with extrahepatic cholestasis in general, but is most characteristic of primary sclerosing cholangitis.
➤ Take a detailed drug history, including prescription drugs, over-the-counter medications, and complementary or herbal remedies.
➤ Family history.
➤ Social history:
  - alcohol
  - illicit drugs
  - intravenous drug abuse and tattoos
  - sexual history
  - occupation and hobbies
  - travel history.

EXAMINATION

➤ General examination:
  - Vital signs (pulse, blood pressure, respiratory rate and temperature).
  - Signs of fulminant hepatic failure include reduced level of consciousness and hepatic flap.
  - Signs of chronic liver disease include clubbing, palmar erythema, spider naevi and gynaecomastia.
  - Cervical lymphadenopathy may occur with pancreatic or biliary tract malignancy.
➤ Abdominal examination:
  - Tenderness in the right upper quadrant may occur with hepatitis, cholecystitis or cholangitis.
  - Hepatomegaly suggests intrinsic liver disease.

Table 20.1 Causes of jaundice

Unconjugated hyperbilirubinaemia

Impaired bilirubin conjugation
- Gilbert's syndrome
- Crigler–Najar syndrome
- Drugs and toxins

Red cell disorders
- Thalassaemias
- Sickle-cell anaemia
- Hereditary spherocytosis
- Hereditary elliptocytosis
- Paroxysmal nocturnal haemoglobinuria
- G6PD deficiency
- Pyruvate kinase deficiency
- Miscellaneous

Autoimmune
- Warm autoimmune haemolytic anaemia
- Cold agglutinin syndrome
- Paroxysmal cold haemoglobinuria
- Drug-induced haemolytic anaemia
- Acute haemolytic transfusion reaction
- Graft-versus-host disease

Microangiopathic
- TTP/HUS
- HELLP syndrome
- Malignant hypertension
- Disseminated intravascular coagulation
- Antiphospholipid syndrome[1]
- Miscellaneous

Mechanical
- Cardiopulmonary bypass
- Metallic heart valve

Intrinsic liver disease

Viral infection
- Hepatitis A or E
- Hepatitis B, C or D
- Epstein–Barr virus
- Cytomegalovirus
- Herpes simplex virus
- Varicella zoster virus
- Adenovirus
- Yellow fever
- Dengue fever
- Viral haemorrhagic fever
- Miscellaneous

Bacterial infection
- Severe sepsis
- Toxic shock syndrome
- Acute appendicitis
- Legionella pneumonia
- Mycoplasma pneumonia
- Pneumococcal pneumonia
- Listeriosis
- Leptospirosis
- Relapsing fever
- Typhoid fever
- Tularaemia
- Lyme disease
- Q fever
- Syphilitic hepatitis
- Miliary tuberculosis
- Visceral leishmaniasis

Disseminated fungal infection
- Cryptococcosis
- Aspergillosis
- Candidiasis
- Miscellaneous

Liver abscess
- Bacterial
- Amoebic
- Hydatid disease

Inflammation
- Alcoholic hepatitis
- Non-alcoholic steatohepatitis
- Autoimmune hepatitis
- Primary biliary cirrhosis
- Haemophagocytic lymphohistiocytosis
- Graft-versus-host disease
- Liver allograft rejection
- Adult Still's disease[3]
- Kawasaki disease[4]

Drugs and toxins
- Paracetamol
- Isoniazid
- Oestrogens
- Halothane
- Herbal medicines
- Hepatotoxic plants
- Amanita mushrooms
- Chlorinated hydrocarbons
- Volatile substance abuse
- Miscellaneous

Vascular
- Ischaemic hepatitis
- Budd–Chiari syndrome
- Veno-occlusive disease
- Portal vein thrombosis
- Septic portal vein thrombophlebitis
- Hepatic artery occlusion

Neoplasia
- Hepatocellular carcinoma
- Hepatic metastases
- Lymphoma
- Leukaemia
- Langerhans cell histiocytosis
- Miscellaneous

Hepatic congestion
- Congestive cardiac failure
- Cor pulmonale
- Constrictive pericarditis
- Restrictive cardiomyopathy
- Tricuspid regurgitation
- Atrial myxoma
- Primary pulmonary hypertension

Pregnancy-related disorders
- Intrahepatic cholestasis of pregnancy
- HELLP syndrome
- Pre-eclampsia
- Eclampsia
- Acute fatty liver of pregnancy
- Hyperemesis gravidarum

Hereditary and congenital
- Haemochromatosis
- Wilson's disease
- α1-antitrypsin deficiency
- Dubin–Johnson syndrome
- Rotor syndrome
- Cystic fibrosis
- Glycogen storage disease
- Gaucher's disease
- Hereditary fructose intolerance
- Tyrosinaemia
- Erythropoietic porphyria
- Progressive familial intrahepatic cholestasis
- Benign recurrent intrahepatic cholestasis
- Hereditary haemorrhagic telangiectasia

Miscellaneous
- Peliosis hepatis
- Nodular regenerative hyperplasia

Extrahepatic cholestasis

Gallstone disease
- Choledocholithiasis
- Cholangitis
- Acute cholecystitis

Pancreatic disease
- Pancreatic cancer
- Acute pancreatitis
- Chronic pancreatitis
- Pancreatic pseudocyst
- Pancreatic tuberculosis

Miscellaneous
- Cholangiocarcinoma
- Primary sclerosing cholangitis
- Secondary sclerosing cholangitis
- Choledochal cyst
- Biliary stricture
- Bile duct trauma
- Haemobilia
- Porta hepatis lymphadenopathy
- Hepatobiliary tuberculosis
- Parasitic infection

Unconjugated hyperbilirubinaemia

▲ Infective endocarditis
▲ Aortic stenosis[2]
▲ March haemoglobinuria

Infection
▲ Malaria
▲ Babesiosis
▲ *Bartonella bacilliformis*
▲ *Clostridium perfringens*
▲ African trypanosomiasis

Miscellaneous
▲ Hypersplenism
▲ Acanthocytosis
▲ Megaloblastic anaemia
▲ Congenital dyserythropoietic anaemia
▲ Hypophosphataemia
▲ Oxidant drugs and toxins
▲ Envenomation

Intrinsic liver disease

Extrahepatic cholestasis

▲ Vanishing bile duct syndrome
▲ Paraneoplastic cholestasis
▲ Amyloidosis[5]
▲ Myelofibrosis
▲ Hyperthyroidism
▲ Total parenteral nutrition
▲ Heat stroke
▲ Radiation hepatitis
▲ Hepatic trauma or surgery

- Splenomegaly may occur in chronic liver disease with portal hypertension, or in conditions associated with extravascular haemolysis, such as red cell membrane disorders, red cell enzymopathies, and haemoglobinopathies.
- Palpable gall-bladder enlargement suggests malignant extrahepatic cholestasis (Courvoisier's sign).
- Ascites suggests chronic liver disease, but may occur with fulminant hepatic failure.
➤ Cardiovascular examination:
  - Signs of systemic venous hypertension, which may cause hepatic congestion, include raised JVP, peripheral oedema and a third heart sound on cardiac auscultation.
  - Right ventricular (left parasternal) heave is a sign of pulmonary hypertension.
  - Kussmaul's sign refers to a JVP that rises on inspiration, rather than falling. It occurs with constrictive pericarditis and restrictive cardiomyopathy.
  - Cardiac auscultation may reveal a pansystolic murmur at the lower left sternal edge, which suggests tricuspid regurgitation.
➤ Miscellaneous findings:
  - Emphysema in association with liver disease suggests α1-antitrypsin deficiency.
  - Movement abnormalities occur with Wilson's disease. Kayser–Fleischer rings may also be seen on examination of the eyes. They are caused by corneal copper deposition.

INVESTIGATIONS

The following core investigations are commonly required:
➤ Blood tests:
  - Bilirubin. The conjugated and unconjugated fractions may also be measured if necessary.
  - LFTs. AST and ALT are disproportionately raised in intrinsic liver disease, whereas ALP is disproportionately raised in extrahepatic cholestasis.
  - Albumin and INR. Hypoalbuminaemia and a raised INR suggest deranged liver synthetic function.
  - FBC. Anaemia suggests haemolysis, whereas a raised WBC occurs with infection.
  - U&Es. Jaundice is often associated with systemic disease such as sepsis that may also cause renal impairment.
  - CRP. Levels are raised with infection and inflammation.
  - Ferritin. Levels are raised in haemochromatosis.
  - Caeruloplasmin. Levels are low in Wilson's disease.
  - α1-Antitrypsin. Levels are low in α1-AT deficiency.
  - Liver autoimmune screen. Anti-smooth muscle and anti-liver/kidney microsomal antibodies are present in autoimmune hepatitis, whereas anti-mitochondrial antibodies occur in primary biliary cirrhosis.
  - Hepatitis A, B and C, EBV and CMV serology.
➤ Pregnancy test.
➤ USS or CT of the abdomen may reveal a variety of structural abnormalities of the liver, biliary tract and pancreas. Examples include gallstone disease, malignancy and biliary tract dilatation.

The following further investigations may be required:
➤ Biochemistry:
  - Amylase. Activity of this enzyme is raised with acute pancreatitis.
  - Lactate dehydrogenase. Activity of this enzyme is raised with haemolysis.
  - Haptoglobin. Levels are low with intravascular haemolysis.
  - TFTs. Hyperthyroidism may cause jaundice.
  - Vitamin B_{12} levels. Pernicious anaemia may cause jaundice.
  - Paracetamol levels.
➤ Haematology:
  - Blood film. Fragmented red cells suggest microangiopathic haemolytic anaemia or mechanical haemolysis. Spherocytes or elliptocytes may be seen with hereditary spherocytosis or elliptocytosis, respectively.
  - Reticulocyte count. This is raised with haemolysis.
  - Thick and thin films are used to diagnose malaria and other red cell parasitoses.
  - Haemoglobinopathy screen.
  - Ham's test. This is positive in paroxysmal nocturnal haemoglobinuria.
  - Direct Coomb's test. This is positive in immune haemolytic anaemias.
➤ Microbiology:
  - Blood culture.
  - Ascitic fluid MC&S may be diagnostic of spontaneous bacterial peritonitis, which is a serious complication of chronic liver disease.
  - HIV test.
  - Lyme serology.
  - Syphilis serology (VDRL or TPHA).
  - Stool microscopy for ova or parasites.

➤ Imaging:
  – ERCP or MRCP is utilised to image the biliary tree and, in the case of ERCP, to perform interventions such as sphincterotomy or gallstone removal.
  – Doppler USS, MRI and formal angiography may be used to assess hepatic arterial or portal vein inflow and hepatic vein outflow.
  – Echocardiogram. Congestive cardiac failure, tricuspid regurgitation or other cardiac abnormalities that cause liver congestion may be detected.
➤ Liver biopsy may be required to diagnose intrinsic liver disease.

REFERENCES

1 Espinosa G, Bucciarelli S, Cervera R *et al*. Thrombotic microangiopathic haemolytic anaemia and antiphospholipid antibodies. *Ann Rheum Dis*. 2004; **63**: 730–6.

2 Kawase I, Matsuo T, Sasayama K *et al*. Haemolytic anaemia with aortic stenosis resolved by urgent aortic valve replacement. *Ann Thorac Surg*. 2008; **86**: 645–6.

3 Dino O, Provanzano G, Giannuoli G *et al*. Fulminant hepatic failure in adult onset Still's disease. *J Rheumatol*. 1996; **23**(4): 784–5.

4 Granel B, Serratrice J, Ene N *et al*. Painful jaundice revealing Kawasaki disease in a young man. *J Gastroenterol Hepatol*. 2004; **19**(6): 713–15.

5 Peters RA, Koukoulis G, Gimson A *et al*. Primary amyloidosis and severe intrahepatic cholestatic jaundice. *Gut*. 1994; **35**(9): 1322–5.

CHAPTER 21

Headache

PATHOPHYSIOLOGY AND AETIOLOGY

Brain tissue itself does not possess pain receptors. Headache therefore arises from the various pain-sensitive structures of the head and neck, namely the meninges, blood vessels, muscles, sinuses, eyes, teeth and gums. Headache, like other forms of pain, may also be neuropathic in origin. Raised intracranial pressure most probably causes headache as a result of traction on the meninges and intracranial blood vessels.

The causes of headache may be conveniently classified into the following five categories:

1. vascular
2. infectious
3. inflammatory
4. miscellaneous
5. extracranial disease.

The causes of headache are listed in Table 21.1, with common causes highlighted in bold type.

EMERGENCY MANAGEMENT

➤ Headache is an extremely common symptom, and although most cases are managed entirely in primary care, a minority represent serious pathology that demands urgent investigation and treatment. The following are examples of important diagnoses that should not be missed:
  – intracranial haemorrhage
  – cerebral venous thrombosis
  – carotid or vertebral artery dissection
  – bacterial or tuberculous meningitis
  – cerebral abscess
  – encephalitis
  – giant-cell arteritis
  – intracranial tumour
  – idiopathic intracranial hypertension
  – pre-eclampsia
  – acute angle-closure glaucoma (AACG).
➤ The following are red flag features that should raise the suspicion of serious underlying pathology. The clinical concern that should be elicited by these features is shown in parentheses:
  – history of head trauma or anticoagulant use (intracranial haemorrhage)
  – instantaneous onset of 'worst ever' headache (subarachnoid haemorrhage)
  – focal weakness or numbness, visual disturbance, ataxia or vertigo (intracranial lesion)
  – papilloedema, reduced level of consciousness, nausea or vomiting (raised intracranial pressure)
  – neck stiffness or photophobia (meningitis or subarachnoid haemorrhage)
  – skin rash (meningococcal meningitis)
  – jaw claudication or scalp tenderness (giant-cell arteritis)
  – ocular pain or erythema (AACG).

HISTORY

➤ Record the mode of onset of the current episode. Instantaneous onset suggests subarachnoid haemorrhage or vascular dissection.

Table 21.1 Causes of headache[1]

Intracranial disease				Extracranial disease
Vascular	*Infection*	*Inflammation*	*Miscellaneous*	
Haemorrhage ▲ Subarachnoid ▲ Subdural ▲ Extradural ▲ Intracerebral ▲ Infratentorial Thromboembolism ▲ Cerebral sinus thrombosis or infection ▲ Ischaemic stroke ▲ Transient ischaemic attack ▲ Pituitary apoplexy Vasculitis ▲ Giant-cell arteritis ▲ Takayasu arteritis ▲ Cerebral vasculitis Vascular trauma ▲ Carotid or vertebral artery dissection ▲ Cerebral vascular intervention Vascular malformations ▲ Arterial aneurysm ▲ Arteriovenous malformation ▲ Cavernous angioma Miscellaneous ▲ Hyperviscosity syndrome ▲ Reversible cerebral vasoconstriction syndrome ▲ CADASIL ▲ MELAS ▲ Degos' disease[2]	Meningitis ▲ Viral meningitis ▲ Pyogenic bacterial meningitis ▲ Tuberculous meningitis ▲ Mycoplama ▲ Legionella ▲ Syphilis ▲ Lyme disease ▲ Brucellosis ▲ Tularaemia ▲ Leptospirosis ▲ Relapsing fever ▲ *Spirillum minus* ▲ Rickettsiosis ▲ Scrub typhus ▲ Ehrlichiosis ▲ Cat scratch disease ▲ Whipple's disease ▲ Fungal meningitis Encephalitis ▲ HSV 1 or 2 ▲ Herpes zoster virus ▲ Epstein–Barr virus ▲ Enteroviruses ▲ West Nile virus ▲ Rabies ▲ PML ▲ HIV ▲ *Listeria monocytogenes* ▲ Miscellaneous Parasitic infection ▲ Malaria ▲ African trypanosomiasis	Aseptic meningitis ▲ Sarcoidosis ▲ Behçet's disease ▲ Systemic lupus erythematosus ▲ Mixed connective tissue disease ▲ Wegener's granulomatosis ▲ Rheumatoid arthritis ▲ Malignant meningitis ▲ Chemical meningitis ▲ Drug-induced meningitis ▲ Vogt-Koyanagi–Harada syndrome ▲ HaNDL ▲ Idiopathic hypertrophic pachymeningitis[3] Miscellaneous ▲ Optic neuritis ▲ Tolosa–Hunt syndrome ▲ Lymphocytic hypophysitis	Primary headache disorders ▲ Tension headache ▲ Migraine ▲ Cluster headache ▲ SUNCT/SUNA ▲ Paroxysmal hemicrania ▲ Hemicrania continua ▲ Miscellaneous Mass lesions ▲ Intracranial tumour ▲ Subdural hygroma Hypertension ▲ Pre-eclampsia ▲ Eclampsia ▲ Malignant hypertension ▲ Sympathomimetic drugs ▲ PRES Cerebral vasodilatation ▲ Hypercapnia ▲ Hypoxia ▲ Sepsis ▲ Hypoglycaemia ▲ Postictal headache ▲ Acute altitude sickness ▲ Hyperperfusion syndrome ▲ Dialysis disequilibrium ▲ Vasodilator drugs ▲ Carbon monoxide CSF pressure abnormalities ▲ Idiopathic intracranial hypertension ▲ Vitamin A toxicity	Acute glaucoma Sinusitis ▲ Viral ▲ Bacterial ▲ Fungal ▲ Allergic Dental disease ▲ Periodontitis ▲ Temporomandibular disorder Cervicogenic headache ▲ Hyperextension injury ▲ Cervical radiculopathy ▲ Miscellaneous Skull disease ▲ Multiple myeloma ▲ Primary bone tumour ▲ Bone metastasis ▲ Osteomyelitis ▲ Mastoiditis ▲ Petrositis ▲ Paget's disease ▲ Osteopetrosis Cardiac ischaemia ▲ Myocardial infarction ▲ Headache angina Neuropathic headache ▲ Shingles ▲ Post-herpetic neuralgia ▲ Trigeminal neuralgia ▲ Miscellaneous

Intracranial disease

Vascular

Infection

➤ Amoebic encephalitis
➤ Toxoplasmosis
➤ Cysticercosis
➤ Hydatid disease
➤ Miscellaneous

Miscellaneous
➤ Intracranial abscess
➤ Bacterial cerebritis
➤ Subdural empyema
➤ Tuberculoma
➤ Intracranial fungal infection

Inflammation

Miscellaneous

➤ Chiari type 1 malformation
➤ CSF leak

Hydrocephalus
➤ Normal-pressure
➤ Communicating
➤ Non-communicating
➤ Congenital

Central headache
➤ Multiple sclerosis
➤ Central post-stroke pain
➤ Hemicrania epileptica

Extracranial disease

Drug-related headache
➤ Medication overuse
➤ Caffeine, opioid or oestrogen
   withdrawal

Hypothroidism

- ➤ Length of history and pattern of symptoms.
- ➤ Site of pain and radiation:
  - – Frontal pain occurs with tension headache and sinusitis.
  - – Temporal location is characteristic of giant-cell arteritis and migraine.
  - – Ocular pain occurs with AACG and cluster headaches.
  - – Occipital headache occurs with subarachnoid haemorrhage and meningitis.
  - – Generalised headache is characteristic of raised intracranial pressure.
- ➤ Character and severity of the pain.
- ➤ Exacerbating or precipitating factors:
  - – Bending or coughing exacerbates the pain of raised intracranial pressure.
  - – Migraine may be exacerbated by light, sound or movement. It may be precipitated by chocolate or other dietary factors.
  - – Headache exacerbated by cough may be due to a Chiari type 1 malformation.
- ➤ Associated symptoms:
  - – Fever suggests infection or inflammation.
  - – Purpuric or petechial skin rash occurs with meningococcal sepsis.
  - – Jaw claudication, scalp tenderness, weight loss and joint or muscle pain are features of giant-cell arteritis.
  - – Nausea and vomiting occur with raised intracranial pressure.
  - – Neck stiffness occurs with meningitis and subarachnoid haemorrhage.
  - – Photophobia is a feature of migraine, meningitis and subarachnoid haemorrhage.
  - – Focal weakness or numbness may occur with intracerebral haemorrhage, ischaemia, tumour or abscess.
  - – Ataxia and vertigo are features of posterior fossa haemorrhage, ischaemia, tumour or abscess.
  - – Visual disturbances occur with migraine, idiopathic intracranial hypertension and AACG.
  - – Ocular pain or erythema occurs with AACG and cavernous sinus thrombosis.
  - – Lacrimation is a feature of cluster headache and other primary neurovascular headaches.
  - – Nasal congestion or discharge occurs with sinusitis, cluster headaches and SUNCT.
  - – Toothache or neck pain may cause a referred headache.
- ➤ Drug history.
- ➤ Social history:
  - – foreign travel
  - – alcohol
  - – illicit drugs
  - – caffeine intake.

EXAMINATION
- ➤ General examination:
  - – Vital signs (pulse, blood pressure, temperature and respiratory rate).
  - – Skin rash may occur with meningococcal sepsis and other systemic infections, vasculitis and collagen vascular disease.
  - – Scalp tenderness or tender non-pulsatile temporal arteries are signs of giant-cell arteritis.
- ➤ Neurological examination:
  - – Glasgow Coma Scale score.
  - – Signs of meningeal irritation include neck stiffness, Kernig's sign (pain elicited by attempting to straighten the knee with the hip flexed) and Brudzinski's sign (flexion of the knee and hip in response to passive flexion of the neck). Meningeal irritation occurs with meningitis or subarachnoid haemorrhage.
  - – Focal neurological signs may allow localisation of an intracranial lesion.
- ➤ Eyes:
  - – Ocular erythema occurs with acute glaucoma and cavernous sinus thrombosis.
  - – Fundoscopy may reveal papilloedema, which is a sign of raised intracranial pressure. Subhyaloid haemorrhage may accompany subarachnoid haemorrhage.
  - – Intra-ocular pressure is raised with acute angle-closure glaucoma.

INVESTIGATIONS
The following core investigations are commonly required:
- ➤ Blood tests:
  - – FBC. A raised WBC suggests infection.
  - – CRP and ESR are raised with any infective or inflammatory process. ESR is particularly useful in the diagnosis of giant-cell arteritis.
- ➤ ECG. Myocardial infarction may rarely present with headache.[4]
- ➤ CT of the brain. This may reveal intracranial haemorrhage, tumour or abscess. However, a normal CT does not completely rule out subarachnoid haemorrhage.

➤ Lumbar puncture. This should *not* be performed if raised intracranial pressure is a possibility, due to the risk of brainstem herniation. A CT or MRI scan of the brain may be required to rule out raised intracranial pressure before proceeding. The following should be assessed:
- Opening pressure.
- Xanthochromia. This is diagnostic of subarachnoid haemorrhage.
- CSF protein and glucose with matched serum glucose
- Cell count. Erythrocytosis may be due to a traumatic tap or subarachnoid haemorrhage. Neutrophilia occurs with bacterial meningitis. Lymphocytosis occurs with tuberculous, syphilitic, fungal or viral meningitis, and with partially treated bacterial meningitis. Eosinophilia occurs with helminth infection.
- MC&S. Consider also performing the Ziehl–Neelsen stain for mycobacteria and India ink stain for cryptococci. Amoebae or helminths may rarely be seen.
- Meningococcal PCR.
- Herpes simplex virus PCR.
- Cytology for malignant cells.

The following further investigations may be required:
➤ Biochemistry:
- TFTs. Hypothyroidism may be associated with headache.
- ANA and anti-dsDNA. These are positive with SLE.
- ABG with COHb level. This should be measured if carbon monoxide poisoning is suspected.
➤ Microbiology:
- Blood culture.
- HIV test.
- Lyme, *Brucella* or syphilis serology.
- Thick and thin films should be reviewed if malaria or trypanosomiasis is a possibility.
➤ Imaging:
- MRI of the brain provides superior imaging of the posterior fossa.
- An MR angiogram may be required to diagnose cerebral venous thrombosis or arterial dissection.
- CT of the sinuses.
- X-ray of the cervical spine.

REFERENCES

1   Headache Classification Subcommittee of the International Headache Society. The International Classification of headache disorders, 2nd edition. *Cephalalgia*. 2004; **24 (Suppl. 1):** 1–160.
2   Caviness VS, Sagar P, Israel EJ *et al*. Case 38-2006: a 5 year old boy with headache and abdominal pain. *NEJM*. 2006; **355:** 2575–84.
3   Kupersmith MJ, Martin V, Heller G *et al*. Idiopathic hypertrophic pachymeningitis. *Neurology*. 2004; **62:** 686–94.
4   Sendovski U, Rabkin Y, Goldshlak L *et al*. Should acute myocardial infarction be considered in the differential diagnosis of headache? *Eur J Emerg Med*. 2009; **16:** 1–3.

CHAPTER 22

Transient loss of consciousness

PATHOPHYSIOLOGY AND AETIOLOGY

Transient loss of consciousness may result from any process that causes sudden reversible cerebral dysfunction. The commonest mechanism for this presentation is a transient drop in cerebral perfusion, known as 'syncope'.

Cardiac causes of syncope include arrhythmias and structural heart diseases such as hypertrophic cardiomyopathy and aortic stenosis. Myocardial infarction may also cause a transient reduction in cardiac output and thus syncope. Non-cardiac causes include vasovagal syncope and carotid sinus hypersensitivity, both of which cause a transient increase in vagus nerve tone, resulting in a sudden reduction in cardiac output. Postural hypotension may result from intravascular volume depletion or from loss of normal orthostatic blood pressure control, due to autonomic neuropathy or drugs (e.g. antihypertensives or vasodilators). Hyperventilation causes syncope by the unique mechanism of inducing hypocapnia and thus cerebral vasoconstriction. Vertebrobasilar ischaemia, subclavian steal syndrome and basilar migraine cause syncope through transient hypoperfusion of the brainstem and thus the reticular activating system.

Transient loss of consciousness may also be caused by impaired delivery of oxygen or glucose to the brain by mechanisms other than reduced perfusion, such as hypoglycaemia, hypoxia and carbon monoxide poisoning. Head injuries and seizures are also common causes of transient loss of consciousness.

The causes of transient loss of consciousness are listed in Table 22.1, with common causes highlighted in bold type.

EMERGENCY MAAGEMENT

➤ Patients with syncope or pre-syncope should immediately be laid flat in order to optimise cerebral perfusion. Failure to do this may result in seizures or permanent neurological damage.
➤ Chest pain, palpitation and exercise-induced syncope are red flags for cardiac disease. Patients with these symptoms require more urgent investigation, often as an inpatient.
➤ Check for evidence of acute haemorrhage in patients with postural hypotension.
➤ Ensure that patients are given appropriate advice about driving, swimming and other activities that are associated with risk in the event of transient loss of consciousness. Patients may be legally obliged to stop driving and to inform the DVLA, depending on their diagnosis. It is the responsibility of doctors to inform patients of this requirement.

HISTORY

➤ Precipitating factors:
  – Exercise-induced syncope occurs with valvular stenosis and hypertrophic cardiomyopathy.
  – Syncope on assuming the upright posture is characteristic of postural hypotension, most commonly due to hypovolaemia or autonomic dysfunction.
  – Emotion, pain, warm environment and prolonged standing are common precipitants of vasovagal syncope.
  – Situational syncope is vasovagal syncope caused by a specific stimulus such as coughing, micturition or defecation. In rare cases, syncope on coughing or sneezing may be due to a Chiari type 1 malformation.
  – Syncope following head movements may occur with carotid sinus hypersensitivity.
➤ Preceding symptoms:
  – Palpitation suggests cardiac arrhythmia.
  – Chest pain may occur with myocardial ischaemia, pulmonary embolism, aortic dissection or cardiac arrhythmia.
  – Anxiety, fast breathing, tingling of the hands or around the mouth, and carpopedal spasm are characteristic of hyperventilation.
  – Dizziness or light-headedness before loss of consciousness commonly occurs with syncope and hypoglycaemia.
  – Vertigo is suggestive of brainstem ischaemia.
  – Absence of preceding symptoms is characteristic of seizure disorders, although in some cases patients may report a variety of curious sensations, particularly with temporal lobe epilepsy.

Table 22.1 Causes of transient loss of consciousness

Syncope		Miscellaneous
Cardiac	*Non-cardiac*	
Cardiac arrhythmia	Hypovolaemia	Head injury
➤ Bradyarrhythmia		
➤ Tachyarrhythmia	Hyperventilation	Seizure
Cardiac outflow obstruction	Autonomic dysfunction	Hypoglycaemia
➤ Hypertrophic cardiomyopathy	➤ Vasovagal syncope	
➤ Aortic stenosis	➤ Carotid sinus hypersensitivity	Carbon monoxide poisoning
➤ Pulmonary stenosis	➤ Autonomic neuropathy	
➤ Mitral or tricuspid stenosis	➤ Vagoglossopharyngeal neuralgia	Asphyxiant gas inhalation
➤ Aortic dissection	➤ Phaeochromocytoma	
➤ Cardiac tamponade	➤ Dopamine β-hydroxylase deficiency	Hypoxia
➤ Atrial myxoma		
➤ Pulmonary embolism	Brainstem ischaemia	Anaemia
➤ Pulmonary hypertension	➤ Vertebrobasilar ischaemia	
	➤ Subclavian steal syndrome	
Myocardial ischaemia	➤ Basilar migraine	
	Drugs	
	➤ Anti-hypertensives	
	➤ Vasodilators	
	➤ Miscellaneous	
	Chiari type 1 malformation	

➤ If the episode was witnessed, ask about the events that occurred while the patient was unconscious. Tongue biting, limb shaking, increased tone and incontinence are characteristic of seizures. However, cerebral hypoperfusion may cause myoclonic jerks, and anoxic seizures can result if a patient with syncope is not immediately laid flat.
➤ Note the speed of recovery. A prolonged phase (more than 30 minutes) of drowsiness or confusion following return of consciousness is characteristic of seizures.
➤ Record the age of onset and the frequency of attacks.
➤ Record the past medical history and drug history.
➤ A family history of syncope suggests a hereditary disorder that predisposes to cardiac arrhythmias, such as a hereditary long-QT syndrome.

EXAMINATION
➤ Vital signs (pulse, blood pressure, respiratory rate, temperature and oxygen saturations).
➤ Perform a general inspection, in particular noting any cyanosis, anaemia or cherry-red skin (seen with severe carbon monoxide poisoning).
➤ Signs of hypovolaemia include tachycardia, tachypnoea, hypotension or postural hypotension, weak thready pulse, cool peripheries, prolonged capillary refill time, dry mucous membranes and reduced skin turgor. Postural hypotension may also be caused by autonomic dysfunction and drugs.
➤ Palpate the pulse. A slow-rising pulse is characteristic of aortic stenosis, whereas hypertrophic cardiomyopathy may give a jerky pulse. An abnormal rate or rhythm suggests an ongoing cardiac arrhythmia.
➤ Assess the jugular venous pressure. It may rise with massive pulmonary embolism or pulmonary hypertension.
➤ Palpate the precordium. Right ventricular heave may occur with massive pulmonary embolism or pulmonary hypertension, whereas a sustained apex beat occurs with severe aortic stenosis.
➤ Auscultate the heart. Systolic murmurs occur with aortic stenosis and hypertrophic cardiomyopathy.
➤ Examine the abdomen, checking in particular for an abdominal aortic aneurysm.
➤ Perform a rectal examination to check for melaena and rectal bleeding.
➤ Perform a full neurological examination. Focal deficits imply a primary neurological condition, although hypoglycaemia, carbon monoxide poisoning and cerebral hypoperfusion of any cause may produce similar findings.

INVESTIGATIONS
The following core investigations are commonly required:
➤ Blood tests:
  – FBC. This may reveal anaemia.

- U&Es, calcium and magnesium. Electrolyte abnormalities may cause arrhythmias.
- Glucose. Hypoglycaemia is a common cause of transient loss of consciousness.
➤ ECG. This may reveal myocardial ischaemia, an ongoing cardiac arrhythmia, or an abnormality that predisposes to arrhythmias, such as Brugada syndrome, pre-excitation, or an abnormally long or short QT interval.
➤ Ambulatory ECG monitoring.

The following further investigations may be required:
➤ ABG with COHb levels.
➤ Troponin I. Levels are raised from 12 hours after myocardial infarction.
➤ D-dimer. Levels are raised with pulmonary embolism.
➤ Tilt-table test. This is used to diagnose disorders of orthostatic blood pressure control.
➤ Echocardiogram. This allows structural heart disease to be visualised.
➤ Cardiac electrophysiological testing. This is used for detailed investigation of cardiac arrhythmias.
➤ EEG. This may provide evidence of a seizure disorder.
➤ CT or MRI of the brain. This may reveal structural abnormalities that predispose to seizures, or a Chiari type 1 malformation.
➤ MR angiogram. This may provide evidence for vertebrobasilar ischaemia or subclavian steal syndrome.

CHAPTER 23

Focal neurological deficit

PATHOPHYSIOLOGY AND AETIOLOGY

When considering the diagnosis of a focal neurological deficit such as limb weakness or numbness, two separate questions must be answered:
1   What is the site of the lesion?
2   What is the nature of the lesion?

The site of the lesion refers to the location of injury within the nervous system (e.g. the L2 level of the spinal cord or the left internal capsule). The nature of the lesion refers to the underlying cause of nervous system injury or dysfunction (e.g. ischaemia, neoplasia or inflammation).

The pattern of weakness or numbness, together with any associated symptoms and signs, will allow clinical localisation of the lesion. In addition, a number of clinical signs may be used to distinguish between upper motor neuron lesions (those that affect the brain and spinal cord) and lower motor neuron lesions (those that affect nerve roots or peripheral nerves), as described below.

Table 23.1 lists the disorders that may affect the brain and spinal cord, while the causes of peripheral neuropathy, neuromuscular junction disease and myopathy are shown in Table 23.2. Nerve root damage (radiculopathy) is most commonly caused by compression within the spinal canal, due to the same pathologies that cause spinal cord compression. However, it is possible for the systemic pathologies that cause peripheral neuropathy to affect a nerve root and thus cause a radiculopathy.

The production of smooth coordinated movements is dependent both on adequate functioning of the cerebellum and on sensory feedback from the joints, muscles and skin. Thus ataxia may be caused by cerebellar disease or by altered sensation (e.g. due to myelopathy or peripheral neuropathy). The extrapyramidal system consists of a number of brain areas such as the nigrostriatal pathway and the basal ganglia that are also involved in the regulation of movement. Extrapyramidal disorders may cause involuntary movements, abnormalities of muscle tone and difficulty in initiating movements. Finally, a small group of conditions are characterised by increased muscle tone without extrapyramidal system involvement. These include tetanus, malignant hyperpyrexia, stiff person syndrome, neuromyotonia and strychnine poisoning. Table 23.3 lists the causes of movement abnormalities due to cerebellar or extrapyramidal disease.

EMERGENCY MANAGEMENT

➤ Patients with acute neuromuscular weakness are at risk of ventilatory failure that may rapidly progress to respiratory arrest. Therefore it is essential to perform an arterial blood gas analysis and monitor the forced vital capacity (FVC) 4- to 6-hourly. An FVC of less than 15 ml/kg of body weight, or less than 1 litre, is an indication for elective intubation and ventilation.[1]
➤ Urgent neurosurgical intervention may be required for a number of conditions, including spinal cord compression, cauda equina syndrome, subarachnoid, subdural or epidural haemorrhage, and massive intracerebral haemorrhage or infarction with mass effect. Significant haemorrhage, infarction, tumour or abscess affecting the posterior fossa is particularly likely to require surgical treatment, due to the possibility of brainstem compression.
➤ Thrombolysis may improve the functional outcome in selected patients with ischaemic stroke if given within three hours of the onset of symptoms and having definitively excluded haemorrhage.[2] Thrombolysis for acute stroke should only be performed in accredited centres by personnel with specialist training.

HISTORY

➤ Time course and onset of symptoms. Sudden onset suggests a vascular event or seizure.
➤ Distribution of weakness or numbness.
➤ Associated symptoms may give an indication of the site of the lesion or its type (indicated in parentheses):
    –   diplopia (brainstem, cranial nerves III, IV or VI, ocular muscles)
    –   dysphasia (cerebral cortex)
    –   dysarthria (cerebellum, brainstem, lower cranial nerves)
    –   dysphagia (brainstem, lower cranial nerves)
    –   vertigo (brainstem, cochlea, vestibular nerve)
    –   back or neck pain (spinal cord or nerve root)

Table 23.1 Causes of brain and spinal cord lesions

Brain

Haemorrhage
➤ Intracerebral
➤ Infratentorial
➤ Subarachnoid
➤ Subdural
➤ Extradural

Thromboembolism
➤ Transient ischaemic attack
➤ Thromboembolic stroke
➤ Cerebral sinus thrombosis
➤ Endocarditis
➤ Atrial myxoma
➤ Cholesterol embolism
➤ Decompression sickness

Vasculitis
➤ Polyarteritis nodosa
➤ Giant-cell arteritis
➤ Wegener's granulomatosis
➤ Churg–Strauss syndrome
➤ Behçet's disease
➤ Primary CNS angiitis
➤ Miscellaneous

Miscellaneous vasculopathy
➤ TTP/HUS
➤ Antiphospholipid syndrome
➤ Sneddon's syndrome
➤ Lymphomatoid granulomatosis
➤ Intravascular lymphoma
➤ Degos' disease
➤ Susac's syndrome
➤ Moyamoya disease
➤ Reversible cerebral vasoconstriction syndrome
➤ Hemiplegic migraine
➤ Fibromuscular dysplasia
➤ Hyperviscosity syndrome
➤ Fabry's disease
➤ CADASIL
➤ PRES

Demyelination
➤ Multiple sclerosis
➤ ADEM
➤ PML
➤ Central pontine myelinolysis
➤ Marchiafava–Bignami disease

Inflammation
➤ Systemic lupus erythematosus
➤ Paraneoplastic encephalomyelitis
➤ Hashimoto's encephalopathy
➤ Rasmussen's encephalitis
➤ VKH syndrome

Infection
➤ **Intracranial abscess**
➤ **Bacterial cerebritis**
➤ **Encephalitis**
➤ Cerebral sinus infection
➤ Tuberculoma
➤ Neurosyphilis
➤ Fungal infection
➤ Malaria
➤ Toxoplasmosis
➤ Helminth infection
➤ Miscellaneous

Neoplasia
➤ **Primary brain tumour**
➤ **Brain metastasis**
➤ **Lymphoma**
➤ Bing–Neel syndrome

Structural
➤ **Hydrocephalus**
➤ Chiari malformation
➤ Syringobulbia
➤ Subdural hygroma
➤ Vascular malformation

Miscellaneous
➤ **Partial seizure**
➤ **Hypoglycaemia**
➤ **Carbon monoxide**
➤ Radiation injury
➤ Cataplexy

Spinal cord

Structural
➤ Trauma
➤ Spondylosis
➤ Spondylolisthesis
➤ Atlantoaxial subluxation
➤ Prolapsed intervertebral disc
➤ Vertebral fracture
➤ Syringomyelia
➤ Spinal dysraphism
➤ Miscellaneous

Neoplasia
➤ **Multiple myeloma**
➤ **Bone metastasis**
➤ Primary bone tumour
➤ Spinal cord tumour
➤ Miscellaneous

Inflammation
➤ **Multiple sclerosis**
➤ Devic's disease
➤ Acute disseminated encephalomyelitis
➤ Systemic lupus erythematosus
➤ Sjögren's syndrome
➤ Neurosarcoidosis
➤ Paraneoplastic necrotising myelopathy
➤ Paraneoplastic encephalomyelitis
➤ Post-infectious transverse myelitis
➤ Radiation myelitis
➤ Spinal pachymeningitis
➤ Miscellaneous

Infection
➤ Vertebral osteomyelitis
➤ Pyogenic discitis
➤ Epidural abscess
➤ Subdural empyema
➤ Intramedullary abscess
➤ Spinal tuberculosis
➤ Neurosyphilis
➤ Lyme disease
➤ Viral myelitis
➤ HIV-associated myelopathy
➤ Tropical spastic paraparesis
➤ Miscellaneous

Vascular
➤ Spinal cord haemorrhage
➤ Epidural haematoma
➤ Subdural haematoma
➤ Superficial siderosis
➤ Spinal cord infarction
➤ Intravascular lymphoma
➤ Cavernous angioma
➤ Arteriovenous malformation
➤ Decompression sickness

Toxic and metabolic
➤ Vitamin B_{12} deficiency
➤ Folate deficiency
➤ Pellagra
➤ Vitamin E deficiency
➤ Copper deficiency
➤ Nitrous oxide
➤ Cyanide poisoning
➤ Lathyrism
➤ Hepatic myelopathy[3]

Hereditary
➤ Hereditary spastic paraparesis
➤ Friedrich's ataxia
➤ Leukodystrophies

- constipation, urinary retention or incontinence (cauda equina syndrome, spinal cord compression, normal-pressure hydrocephalus, midline anterior cerebral lesion)
- dyspnoea (neuromuscular weakness)
- muscle pain (myopathy).

➤ Dietary history may reveal evidence of vitamin deficiency, botulism or poisoning with marine neurotoxins.

➤ Past medical history. This includes stroke risk factors such as hypertension, dyslipidaemia and atrial fibrillation.

➤ Drug history. Acute neurological deficit in a patient taking anticoagulants mandates urgent brain imaging to diagnose or rule out intracranial haemorrhage.

Table 23.2 Causes of peripheral neuropathy, neuromuscular junction disease and myopathy

Peripheral neuropathy

Motor neuron disease

Structural damage
- Traumatic nerve injury
- Compression neuropathy
- Cauda equina syndrome

Infection
- Herpes zoster
- Poliomyelitis
- Hepatitis B
- HIV
- West Nile virus
- Tick-borne encephalitis
- Diphtheria
- Lyme disease
- Leprosy
- Meningitis

Endocrine and metabolic
- Diabetes mellitus
- Chronic renal failure
- Amyloidosis
- Hypothyroidism
- Acromegaly
- Sarcoidosis
- Acute porphyria
- Chronic liver disease

Nutrient deficiency
- Vitamin B_{12}
- Pyridoxine
- Thiamine (beriberi)
- Niacin (pellagra)
- Vitamin E
- Copper

Electrolyte and acid–base disorders
- Hypocapnia
- Hypocalcaemia
- Hyperkalaemia

Drugs and toxins
- Alcohol
- Lead
- Isoniazid
- Ethambutol
- Vinca alkaloids
- Platinum chemotherapy
- NRTIs
- Miscellaneous

Ischaemia and necrosis
- Acute limb ischaemia
- Compartment syndrome
- Frostbite
- Buerger's disease
- Raynaud's syndrome
- Cold agglutinin disease

Immune-mediated
- Guillain–Barré syndrome
- CIDP
- Paraneoplastic neuropathy
- Paraproteinaemic neuropathy
- POEMS syndrome
- CANOMAD syndrome
- Multifocal motor neuropathy
- Post-infectious neuropathy
- Post-asthmatic amyotrophy[4]
- Miscellaneous

Vasculitis
- Polyarteritis nodosa
- Microscopic polyangiitis
- Churg–Strauss syndrome
- Wegener's granulomatosis
- Behçet's disease
- Cryoglobulinaemia
- Serum sickness
- Non-systemic vasculitic neuropathy
- Paraneoplastic vasculitic neuropathy

Connective tissue disease
- Systemic lupus erythematosus
- Mixed connective tissue disease
- Sjögren's syndrome
- Systemic sclerosis
- Rheumatoid arthritis

Hereditary
- Charcot–Marie–Tooth disease
- Fabry's disease
- Miscellaneous

Miscellaneous
- Bell's palsy
- Neuralgic amyotrophy
- Idiopathic lumbosacral plexus neuropathy
- Critical illness polyneuropathy
- Radiation neuropathy
- Eosinophilia-myalgia syndrome
- Neurolymphomatosis
- Peripheral nerve tumours

Neuromuscular junction and muscle disorders

Neuromuscular blockade
- Myasthenia gravis
- LEMS
- Botulism
- Marine neurotoxins
- Tick paralysis
- Envenomation
- Organophosphates
- Congenital myasthenic syndromes

Inflammatory and autoimmune
- Polymyositis
- Dermatomyositis
- Inclusion body myositis
- Systemic lupus erythematosus
- Systemic sclerosis
- Mixed connective tissue disease
- Sjögren's syndrome
- Rheumatoid arthritis
- Polyarteritis nodosa
- Paraneoplastic necrotising myopathy

Endocrine, toxic and metabolic
- Alcoholic myopathy
- Drug-induced myopathy
- Cushing's syndrome
- Vitamin D deficiency
- Hyperparathyroidism
- Adrenal insufficiency
- Hypo/hyperthyroidism
- Acromegaly
- Diabetic amyotrophy
- Amyloid myopathy
- Carcinoid syndrome
- Rhabdomyolysis

Electrolyte disorders
- Hypo/hypercalcaemia
- Hypo/hyperkalaemia
- Hypophosphataemia
- Hypo/hypermagnesaemia

Infectious myositis
- HIV
- HTLV-1
- Influenza
- Enteroviruses
- Lyme disease
- Tuberculosis
- Toxoplasmosis
- Chagas' disease
- Trichinosis
- Miscellaneous

Inherited myopathies
- Muscular dystrophy
- Myotonic dystrophy
- Congenital myopathies
- Myotonia congenita
- Paramyotonia congenita
- Periodic paralyses
- Slow channel syndrome
- Inborn errors of metabolism
- Mitochondrial encephalomyopathies
- Miscellaneous

Ischaemia and necrosis
- Acute limb ischaemia
- Compartment syndrome
- Frostbite

Table 23.3 Causes of movement abnormalities due to cerebellar or extrapyramidal disease

Cerebellar

Toxic, endocrine and metabolic
➤ Alcohol
➤ Phenytoin
➤ Lithium
➤ Wernicke's encephalopathy
➤ Vitamin E deficiency
➤ Hypothyroidism[5]

Vascular
➤ Cerebellar haemorrhage
➤ Thromboembolic stroke
➤ Vertebrobasilar insufficiency
➤ Subclavian steal syndrome
➤ Basilar migraine
➤ Hyperviscosity syndrome
➤ Superficial siderosis
➤ Miscellaneous

Demyelination
➤ Multiple sclerosis
➤ Acute disseminated
  encephalomyelitis
➤ Progressive multifocal
  leukoencephalopathy

Space-occupying lesions
➤ Tumour
➤ Abscess
➤ Tuberculoma
➤ Miscellaneous

Structural abnormalities
➤ Chiari malformation
➤ Dandy-Walker syndrome

Autoimmune
➤ Paraneoplastic cerebellar
  degeneration
➤ Opsoclonus–myoclonus syndrome
➤ Gluten ataxia[6]
➤ Hashimoto's thyroiditis[7]
➤ Acute cerebellar ataxia
➤ Miller–Fisher syndrome

Hereditary
➤ Friedrich's ataxia
➤ Spinocerebellar ataxias
➤ Episodic ataxias
➤ Leukodystrophies
➤ Ataxia telangiectasia
➤ Miscellaneous

Miscellaneous
➤ Multiple system atrophy
➤ Viral encephalitis
➤ Bacterial cerebellitis
➤ Idiopathic hypertrophic
  pachymeningitis[8]
➤ Prion disease
➤ Heatstroke
➤ Altitude sickness

Extrapyramidal

Acquired neurodegenerative diseases
➤ Parkinson's disease
➤ Multiple system atrophy
➤ Progressive supranuclear palsy
➤ Lewy body disease
➤ Corticobasal degeneration
➤ Chronic hepatocerebral
  degeneration
➤ Neuronal intranuclear inclusion
  disease
➤ Neurodegeneration with brain iron
  accumulation
➤ Neuroferritinopathy
➤ Basal ganglia calcification

Vascular
➤ Intracerebral haemorrhage
➤ Cerebrovascular disease
➤ Hyperviscosity syndrome
➤ Arteriovenous malformation
➤ Miscellaneous

Drug reactions
➤ Drug-induced parkinsonism
➤ Drug-induced chorea
➤ Neuroleptic malignant syndrome
➤ Tardive dyskinesia
➤ Tardive dystonia
➤ Acute dystonia
➤ Miscellaneous

Toxins
➤ MPTP
➤ Methanol
➤ Manganese
➤ Mercury
➤ Wasp sting[9]

Hereditary
➤ Huntington's chorea
➤ Wilson's disease
➤ Acaeruloplasminaemia
➤ Neuroacanthocytosis
➤ Dentatorubropallidoluysian atrophy
➤ Lysosomal disorders
➤ Leukodystrophies
➤ Mitochondrial
  encephalomyopathies
➤ Inborn errors of metabolism
➤ Benign hereditary chorea
➤ Hereditary dystonias
➤ Miscellaneous

Autoimmune and inflammatory
➤ Systemic lupus erythematosus
➤ Antiphospholipid syndrome
➤ Rheumatic chorea
➤ Paraneoplastic chorea,
  parkinsonism or myoclonus[10]
➤ Hashimoto's encephalopathy

Space-occupying lesions
➤ Tumour
➤ Abscess
➤ Miscellaneous

Miscellaneous
➤ Head injury
➤ Cerebral palsy
➤ Post-anoxic encephalopathy
➤ HSV encephalitis
➤ Subacute sclerosing
  panencephalitis
➤ Prion disease
➤ Hyperthyroidism

➤ Family history. This should focus on inherited neurological disorders.
➤ Alcohol intake and use of illicit drugs.

EXAMINATION

➤ Speech. Note expressive or receptive dysphasia (cortical lesion) or dysarthria (cerebellar disease, bulbar palsy or pseudobulbar palsy).
➤ Extrapyramidal disorders may cause involuntary movements such as tremor, myoclonus, chorea, hemiballismus and tics. Bradykinesia (slow movement) and an expressionless face may also be seen.
➤ Gait:
  - Shuffling gait with difficulty starting and stopping occurs with parkinsonism.
  - Broad-based gait is characteristic of cerebellar ataxia, whereas stamping gait is a feature of sensory ataxia.
  - Romberg's test is positive if the patient is able to maintain balance with the feet together if the eyes are open but not if the eyes are closed. The examiner should be ready to catch the patient while performing this test. A positive Romberg's test is a sign of sensory ataxia.
➤ Eyes:
  - Check pupillary reflexes to light and accommodation.
  - Ptosis may be due to neuromuscular weakness or a cranial nerve III palsy.
  - Nystagmus occurs with vestibular or cerebellar disease.
  - Examine the visual fields:
    a Retinal lesions produce a scotoma, which is central if the macula is involved.
    b Optic nerve lesions cause monocular visual loss.
    c Lesions at the optic chiasm cause bitemporal hemianopia.
    d Optic tract lesions cause homonymous hemianopia without macular sparing.
    e Lesions of the temporal or parietal components of the optic radiation cause a homonymous upper or lower quadrantanopia, respectively.
    f Lesions of the occipital cortex cause homonymous hemianopia with macular sparing.
  - Check eye movements. Note that raised intracranial pressure of any cause may produce a cranial nerve VI palsy.
  - Perform fundoscopy. Papilloedema is a feature of raised intracranial pressure.
➤ Facial movement and sensation:
  - Check the corneal reflex bilaterally.
  - Facial numbness may be due to a contralateral cerebral hemisphere lesion or damage to the ipsilateral cranial nerve V or cranial nerve V sensory nucleus in the pons.
  - Unilateral facial weakness with sparing of the upper face results from lesions of the contralateral cerebral hemisphere or corticobulbar tract. Facial weakness without sparing of the upper face is caused by lower motor neuron lesions of cranial nerve VII.
➤ Lower cranial nerves:
  - Check the gag reflex bilaterally (cranial nerves IX and X).
  - Test palatal (cranial nerve X) and tongue (cranial nerve XII) movement.
  - Test shoulder elevation and lateral head rotation (cranial nerve XI).
➤ Inspect the limbs. Muscle wasting or fasciculation occurs with lower motor neuron lesions.
➤ Perform the straight leg raise test. The test is positive if pain radiating down the lower limb in a sciatic nerve distribution is elicited by elevating the limb straight off the bed between 30 and 70 degrees. The crossed straight leg raise is positive if the same manoeuvre causes pain in the opposite leg. If either test is positive, cauda equina syndrome should be suspected and an urgent MRI of the spine should be arranged.
➤ Check power in all muscle groups. The distribution of any weakness suggests the likely site of the lesion or its type:[11]
  - Proximal weakness occurs with myopathies, whereas distal weakness may occur with a generalised peripheral neuropathy.
  - Weakness of the muscles innervated by a specific nerve (e.g. the radial nerve) suggests a mononeuropathy.
  - Muscle weakness affecting a particular myotome occurs with nerve root pathology, whereas damage to all or part of the brachial or lumbosacral plexi may cause weakness that affects a number of adjacent myotomes.
  - Paraplegia is caused by midline anterior cerebral lesions, hydrocephalus, low spinal cord lesions or cauda equina syndrome.
  - Tetraplegia occurs with high spinal cord or brainstem lesions.
  - Hemiplegia is caused by contralateral cerebral hemisphere or brainstem lesions, or ipsilateral cervical spinal cord lesions.
  - Less extensive lesions of the contralateral cerebral hemisphere or brainstem may cause weakness of a single upper or lower limb only, whereas a unilateral thoracic or lumbar spinal cord lesion may cause weakness of the ipsilateral lower limb in isolation.

➤ Check tone, reflexes and coordination in all four limbs:
 - Tone is generally reduced with lower motor neuron lesions and increased with upper motor neuron lesions. However, spinal cord injury causes reduced tone initially, followed by the development of spasticity over the next few days. Cogwheel or lead-pipe rigidity occurs with Parkinson's disease and other extrapyramidal disorders.
 - Reflexes are sluggish or absent with lower motor neuron lesions and brisk with upper motor neuron lesions, except immediately after spinal cord injury. Each tendon reflex tests the function of a particular peripheral nerve and spinal cord level, as follows:
   a   biceps (musculocutaneous nerve, C5–6)
   b   supinator (radial nerve, C6–7)
   c   triceps (radial nerve, C6–8)
   d   knee (femoral nerve, L2–4)
   e   ankle (sciatic nerve, S1–2).
 - Check the plantar responses. An extensor response suggests an upper motor neuron lesion.
 - Test coordination in the upper limbs by using the finger–nose test or by asking the patient to rapidly pronate and supinate their wrist. In the lower limbs use the heel–shin test. Impaired coordination is a sign of cerebellar disease.
➤ Check the major sensory modalities, namely light touch, pin-prick, vibration sense and joint position sense. The distribution of any sensory deficit suggests the site or type of lesion.[11]
 - Glove and/or stocking distribution is characteristic of peripheral neuropathy.
 - Sensory loss within the area innervated by a specific nerve (e.g. the ulnar nerve) suggests a mononeuropathy.
 - Dermatomal distribution occurs with nerve root pathology. Damage to part or all of the brachial or lumbosacral plexi may cause sensory loss within a number of adjacent dermatomes.
 - Sensory level (loss of pain and light touch sensation in all dermatomes below a particular level) occurs as a result of a contralateral spinal cord lesion. Vibration sense and joint position sense may be lost on the side ipsilateral to the lesion. A bilateral spinal cord lesion will cause bilateral sensory loss that affects all modalities.
 - Central spinal cord lesions such as syringomyelia may cause a sensory level with sacral sparing.
 - Hemisensory loss may be caused by damage to the contralateral cerebral hemisphere or brainstem. A less extensive lesion may cause sensory loss in a single limb.
 - Sensory loss within the saddle region suggests cauda equina syndrome or anterior spinal cord damage.
➤ Perform a rectal examination if indicated. Loss of anal tone or perianal sensation occurs with cauda equina syndrome.

INVESTIGATIONS

The following core investigations are commonly required:
➤ Blood tests:
 - FBC and CRP. Raised WBC or CRP indicates infection or inflammation.
 - Glucose and lipid profile. Risk factors for thromboembolic stroke include diabetes mellitus and hyperlipidaemia.
 - U&Es and calcium. Electrolyte abnormalities may cause generalised muscle weakness.
➤ Imaging:
 - CT of the brain. This is the most widely available imaging modality.
 - MRI of the brain. This provides better imaging of the posterior fossa than CT.
 - MRI of the spine.
 - CT or MR angiogram. This should be performed if vascular pathology such as arterial dissection is suspected.

The following further investigations may be required:
➤ In cases of neuromuscular weakness (e.g. due to Guillain–Barré syndrome), an arterial blood gas analysis and regular forced vital capacity measurements are essential in order to detect incipient ventilatory failure.
➤ Biochemistry:
 - TFTs. Thyroid dysfunction may result in myopathy.
 - Vitamin B_{12} and folic acid levels. Deficiencies may result in myelopathy.
 - Serum ACE. Levels may be raised with neurosarcoidosis.
 - Serum electrophoresis and free light chains and urinary Bence Jones protein. These may be diagnostic of plasma cell dyscrasias such as multiple myeloma.
➤ Connective tissue disease and vasculitis screen:
 - ANA and anti-dsDNA (SLE)
 - RhF (rheumatoid arthritis)
 - anti-Ro and anti-La (Sjögren's syndrome)
 - anti-Jo-1 (polymyositis and dermatomyositis)

- – anti-RNP (mixed connective tissue disease)
- – Scl-70 and anticentromere antibodies (systemic sclerosis)
- – ANCA (Churg–Strauss syndrome and Wegener's granulomatosis)
- – anti-cardiolipin antibodies and lupus anticoagulant (antiphospholipid syndrome).
➤ Miscellaneous autoantibodies:
- – tissue transglutaminase and anti-endomysial antibodies (gluten ataxia)
- – anti-GAD antibodies (stiff person syndrome)
- – anti-Yo and anti-Hu antibodies (paraneoplastic cerebellar degeneration or opsoclonus–myoclonus syndrome)
- – anti-AChR and anti-MuSK antibodies (myasthenia gravis).
➤ Serology:
- – CMV, HIV and HTLV-1
- – syphilis
- – Lyme disease
- – *Toxoplasma*.
➤ Lumbar puncture. This should **not** be performed if raised intracranial pressure is a possibility, due to the risk of brainstem herniation. A CT or MRI scan of the brain may be required in order to rule out raised intracranial pressure before proceeding. The following tests may be performed, depending on the clinical picture:
- – Xanthochromia is diagnostic of subarachnoid haemorrhage.
- – CSF protein and glucose with matched serum glucose. CSF protein may be raised with Guillain–Barré syndrome, whereas CSF glucose is reduced with some meningitides.
- – Electrophoresis. Oligoclonal bands occur with multiple sclerosis.
- – Cell count. Erythrocytosis occurs with a traumatic tap or subarachnoid haemorrhage. Neutrophilia is a feature of bacterial meningitis, whereas lymphocytosis occurs with tuberculous, syphilitic, fungal or viral meningitis, as well as with partially treated bacterial meningitis.
- – Microscopy and culture, Gram stain for bacteria, Ziehl–Neelsen stain for mycobacteria, and India ink stain for cryptococci.
- – Meningococcal or HSV PCR.
➤ Miscellaneous tests:
- – Muscle biopsy may be required for the diagnosis of myopathy or myositis.
- – The Tensilon test is used to diagnose myasthenia gravis.
- – Nerve conduction studies may be helpful to confirm peripheral neuropathy.
- – Electroencephalogram may show evidence of seizure activity.
- – Carotid Doppler is performed in cases of anterior circulation thromboembolic stroke to look for carotid artery stenosis that may be amenable to surgical correction.
- – Echocardiogram is performed in cases of thromboembolic stroke to diagnose cardiac sources of emboli.

REFERENCES

1   Ramrakha P, Moore K. *Oxford Handbook of Acute Medicine*. 2nd ed. Oxford: Oxford University Press; 2007. p. 504.
2   Intercollegiate Stroke Working Party. *National Clinical Guidelines for Stroke*. 2nd ed. London: Royal College of Physicians; 2004. p. 35.
3   Yin YH, Ma ZJ, Guan YH et al. Clinical features of hepatic myelopathy in patients with chronic liver disease. *Postgrad Med J*. 2009; **85**: 64–8.
4   Liedholm LJ, Eeg-Olofsson O, Ekenberg BE et al. Acute postasthmatic amyotrophy (Hopkins' syndrome). *Muscle Nerve*. 1994; **17**(7): 769–72.
5   Mistry N, Wass J, Turner MR. When to consider thyroid dysfunction in the neurology clinic. *Pract Neurol*. 2009; 9: 145–56.
6   Hadjivassilou M, Grunewald R, Sharrak B et al. Gluten ataxia in perspective: epidemiology, genetic susceptibility and clinical characteristics. *Brain*. 2003; **126**: 685–91.
7   Selim M, Drachman DA. Ataxia associated with Hashimoto's disease: progressive non-familial adult-onset cerebellar degeneration with autoimmune thyroiditis. *J Neurol Neurosurg Psychiatry*. 2001; **71**: 81–7.
8   Kupersmith MJ, Martin V, Heller G et al. Idiopathic hypertrophic pachymeningitis. *Neurology*. 2004; **62**: 686–94.
9   Leopold NA, Bara-Jimenez W, Hallett M. Parkinsonism after a wasp sting. *Movement Disord*. 2001; **14**: 122–7.
10   Mehta SH, Morgan JC, Sethi KD. Paraneoplastic movement disorders. *Curr Neurol Neurosci Rep*. 2009; **9**(4): 285–91.
11   Lindsay KW, Bone I. *Neurology and Neurosurgery Illustrated*. 3rd ed. New York: Churchill Livingstone; 1997. pp. 191–9.

CHAPTER 24

Acute visual loss

PATHOPHYSIOLOGY AND AETIOLOGY

Visual loss may be caused by pathology affecting any part of the neurological pathway comprising the eye, optic nerve, optic chiasm, optic tract, optic radiation and occipital cortex. Disruption of this pathway may result in visual field defects, reduced visual acuity or complete visual loss. The commonest ocular causes of acute visual loss are acute angle-closure glaucoma (AACG), retinal vascular occlusion, retinal detachment, and preretinal or vitreous haemorrhage. The optic nerve is commonly affected by ischaemia, demyelination and drug toxicity. The optic chiasm lies adjacent to the pituitary gland, and thus pituitary and suprasellar tumours often result in bitemporal hemianopia, due to impingement on the central fibres that are crossing over at this site. The optic tract, optic radiation and occipital cortex are vulnerable to any of the pathologies that may affect the cerebral hemispheres in general, including ischaemia, haemorrhage, neoplasia and demyelination.

The causes of acute visual loss are listed in Table 24.1, with common causes highlighted in bold type. It should be noted that patients may occasionally report sudden monocular visual loss when in fact the deficit has been long-standing but was not previously noticed.

EMERGENCY MANAGEMENT

Treatment will depend on the underlying cause of visual loss. The following are examples of conditions that require urgent treatment:

➤ Giant-cell arteritis. This requires high-dose corticosteroids.
➤ AACG. Urgent referral to an ophthalmologist is mandatory. Initial treatment includes IV acetazolamide, topical β-blockers and topical steroids.
➤ Retinal detachment, vitreous haemorrhage and retinal artery occlusion are also conditions in which time is of the essence. Urgent referral to an ophthalmologist is indicated for consideration of surgical or other treatment that may be sight-saving.

HISTORY

➤ Presenting complaint. Note whether the visual loss affects one or both eyes.
➤ Speed of onset and time course of symptoms. Sudden onset of visual loss suggests optic neuritis, retinal detachment or a vascular event, and subsequent spontaneous resolution would be most characteristic of amaurosis fugax.
➤ Associated symptoms:
  – Ocular pain and erythema suggest AACG, whereas pain alone occurs with optic neuritis.
  – Headache is a feature of giant-cell arteritis, raised intracranial pressure, pituitary gland enlargement and AACG, whereas scalp tenderness and jaw claudication are specific features of giant-cell arteritis.
  – Weakness or altered sensation suggests a cerebral lesion.
➤ Drug history.
➤ Family history.
➤ Smoking and alcohol intake.

EXAMINATION

➤ General examination:
  – Blood pressure. Hypertension predisposes to acute ischaemic and haemorrhagic events, as well as to hypertensive retinopathy.
  – Tender non-pulsatile temporal arteries occur with giant-cell arteritis.
  – Cushingoid or acromegalic appearance suggests a hormone-producing pituitary adenoma.
➤ Inspection of the eye. Ocular erythema occurs with AACG and keratitis.
➤ Visual acuity. This should be checked using a Snellen chart.
➤ Visual fields. The nature of the visual field defect may indicate the site of pathology:
  – Retinal lesions produce a scotoma, which is central if the macula is involved.
  – Optic nerve lesions cause monocular visual loss.
  – Lesions at the optic chiasm cause bitemporal hemianopia.
  – Optic tract lesions cause homonymous hemianopia without macular sparing.

Table 24.1 Causes of acute visual loss

Eye	Optic nerve	Brain
Keratitis	Ischaemia ➤ Amaurosis fugax ➤ Giant-cell arteritis ➤ Non-arteritic ischaemic optic neuropathy	Optic chiasm compression ➤ Pituitary adenoma ➤ Suprasellar tumour ➤ Cerebral aneurysm ➤ Pituitary apoplexy ➤ Lymphocytic hypophysitis
Posterior scleritis		
Uveitis		
Anterior chamber disease ➤ Acute angle-closure glaucoma ➤ Hypopyon ➤ Hyphaemia	Optic neuritis ➤ Multiple sclerosis ➤ Isolated optic neuritis ➤ ADEM ➤ Devic's disease ➤ Parainfectious ➤ Sarcoidosis ➤ Syphilis ➤ Lyme disease ➤ Cryptococcal meningitis ➤ Miscellaneous	Vascular ➤ Intracranial haemorrhage ➤ Transient ischaemic attack ➤ Thromboembolic stroke ➤ Cerebral venous thrombosis ➤ Miscellaneous
Intra-ocular disease ➤ Bacterial endophthalmitis ➤ Fungal endophthalmitis ➤ Vitreous haemorrhage ➤ Foreign body ➤ Trauma		Demyelination ➤ Multiple sclerosis ➤ ADEM ➤ PML ➤ Leukodystrophies
Retinal vascular disease ➤ Amaurosis fugax ➤ Retinal artery occlusion ➤ Retinal vein occlusion ➤ Preretinal haemorrhage ➤ Ocular ischaemic syndrome ➤ Purtscher retinopathy ➤ Hyperviscosity syndrome ➤ Retinal migraine ➤ Susac's syndrome	Raised intracranial pressure ➤ Idiopathic intracranial hypertension ➤ Intracranial tumour ➤ Obstructive hydrocephalus ➤ Miscellaneous	Space-occupying lesion ➤ Tumour ➤ Abscess ➤ Arteriovenous malformation ➤ Miscellaneous
Structural disorders ➤ Retinal detachment ➤ Retinal pigment epithelium detachment	Orbital disease ➤ Thyroid eye disease ➤ Tolosa-Hunt syndrome ➤ Idiopathic orbital inflammatory disease ➤ Wegener's granulomatosis ➤ Langerhans cell histiocytosis ➤ Sarcoidosis ➤ Orbital cellulitis ➤ Mucormycosis ➤ Aspergillosis ➤ Tumour ➤ Fibrous dysplasia	Miscellaneous ➤ Hypoglycaemia ➤ Carbon monoxide poisoning ➤ Radiation encephalopathy ➤ Partial seizure ➤ Posterior reversible encephalopathy syndrome ➤ Bacterial cerebritis ➤ Rasmussen's encephalitis ➤ MELAS ➤ Prion disease
Infectious retinitis ➤ Cytomegalovirus ➤ Herpes simplex ➤ Varicella zoster ➤ Toxoplasmosis ➤ Toxocariasis ➤ Cysticercosis ➤ Diffuse unilateral subacute neuroretinitis		
	Drugs and toxins ➤ Ethambutol ➤ Isoniazid ➤ Quinine ➤ Amiodarone ➤ Methanol ➤ Ethylene glycol ➤ Miscellaneous	
Miscellaneous retinopathies ➤ Central serous ➤ Paraneoplastic ➤ Autoimmune ➤ Leukaemic ➤ Drug-induced ➤ Radiation ➤ Solar	Miscellaneous ➤ Vitamin B_{12} deficiency ➤ Leber's hereditary optic neuropathy ➤ Idiopathic hypertrophic pachymeningitis[1] ➤ Leukaemia ➤ Irradiation ➤ Trauma	

- Lesions of the temporal or parietal components of the optic radiation cause a homonymous upper or lower quadrantanopia, respectively.
- Lesions of the occipital cortex cause homonymous hemianopia with macular sparing.
➤ Fundoscopy and slit lamp examination.
➤ Check the intra-ocular pressure, which is raised with AACG.
➤ Perform a full neurological examination. Associated focal neurological deficits, such as weakness or altered sensation, suggest a CNS disorder.

INVESTIGATIONS

The following core investigations are commonly required:

➤ Blood tests:
- ESR. This is increased with infection or inflammation, and is particularly useful in the diagnosis of giant-cell arteritis.
- CRP. This is raised with infection or inflammation.
- FBC. Polycythaemia or thrombocytosis may predispose to amaurosis fugax.
- Glucose and lipid profile. Diabetes and hyperlipidaemia predispose to thromboembolic stroke, transient ischaemic attacks and amaurosis fugax. Chronic hyperglycaemia leads to diabetic retinopathy.

➤ CT or MRI of the brain is required if CNS pathology is suspected.

The following further investigations may be required:

➤ Blood tests:
- Plasma viscosity. This should be measured if hyperviscosity syndrome is suspected.
- Vitamin B_{12}. Deficiency may cause optic neuropathy.
- Syphilis and Lyme disease serology.

➤ Temporal artery biopsy. This should be performed if giant-cell arteritis is suspected.

➤ Lumbar puncture. Opening pressure is raised with idiopathic intracranial hypertension. Before undertaking lumbar puncture in a patient with papilloedema or other signs of raised intracranial pressure, it is essential to perform a CT or MRI of the head in order to rule out space-occupying lesions, due to the risk of fatal brainstem herniation. Lumbar puncture should only be performed after consultation with a senior clinician.

➤ Miscellaneous tests:
- Carotid Doppler should be performed in order to detect carotid stenosis in cases of amaurosis fugax and ischaemic strokes.
- Echocardiogram should be performed in cases of ischaemic stroke or amaurosis fugax in order to detect left atrial thrombus, atrial myxoma or infective endocarditis.

REFERENCE

1   Kupersmith MJ, Martin V, Heller G *et al*. Idiopathic hypertrophic pachymeningitis. *Neurology*. 2004; **62**: 686–94.

CHAPTER 25

Vertigo

PATHOPHYSIOLOGY AND AETIOLOGY

True vertigo is a sensation that the patient or his or her surroundings are rotating. It should be distinguished from 'light-headedness' or pre-syncope. Dizziness is a non-specific term that should be further clarified before pursuing a differential diagnosis.

The perception of linear or rotatory acceleration is one of the functions of the vestibular system, which comprises the vestibular apparatus of the inner ear, the vestibular nerve and the brainstem. Vertigo may be caused by dysfunction of any of these components. The causes of vertigo are listed in Table 25.1, with common causes highlighted in bold type.

Table 25.1 Causes of vertigo

Central	Peripheral
Vascular	Vestibular nerve disorders
➤ **Posterior fossa haemorrhage**	➤ **Vestibular neuritis**
➤ **Brainstem infarction**	➤ **Ramsay Hunt syndrome**
➤ **Vertebrobasilar insufficiency**	➤ Vestibular paroxysmia
➤ Subclavian steal syndrome	➤ Mononeuritis multiplex
➤ Vertebral artery dissection	➤ Neurosarcoidosis
➤ Vertebrobasilar dolichoectasia	➤ Lyme disease
➤ Takayasu arteritis	➤ Tuberculous meningitis
➤ Cerebral vasculitis	➤ Miscellaneous meningitides
➤ Intravascular lymphoma	
➤ Basilar migraine	Structural cochlear disorders
➤ Hyperviscosity syndrome	➤ **Benign paroxysmal positional vertigo**
	➤ **Ménière's disease**
Space-occupying lesions	➤ **Perilymph fistula**
➤ **Vestibular schwannoma**	➤ Otosclerosis
➤ Meningioma	➤ Cholesteatoma
➤ Brainstem abscess	➤ Temporal bone fracture
➤ Miscellaneous	➤ Superior canal dehiscence syndrome[1]
	➤ Barotrauma
Inflammation/demyelination	
➤ **Multiple sclerosis**	Labyrinthitis
➤ Acute disseminated encephalomyelitis	➤ **Viral**
➤ Progressive multifocal leukoencephalopathy	➤ Bacterial
➤ Paraneoplastic brainstem encephalitis	➤ Syphilis
	➤ Radiation
Toxic/metabolic	
➤ **Ethanol intoxication**	Ototoxic drugs
➤ Wernicke's encephalopathy	➤ Aminoglycosides
➤ Hypomagnesaemia	➤ Loop diuretics
	➤ Carboplatin
Structural	➤ Cisplatin
➤ Chiari malformation	➤ Miscellaneous
➤ Syringobulbia	
➤ Trauma	Autoimmune inner ear disease
	➤ Cogan's syndrome
Miscellaneous	➤ Susac's syndrome
➤ Psychogenic vertigo	➤ Vogt–Koyanagi–Harada syndrome
➤ Central positional vertigo	➤ Miscellaneous
➤ Vertiginous seizure	
➤ Episodic ataxia	

EMERGENCY MANAGEMENT

➤ Although many cases of acute vertigo are caused by relatively benign peripheral disorders, such as vestibular neuritis or benign paroxysmal positional vertigo, it is important to diagnose serious central causes, such as neoplasia, haemorrhage or ischaemia affecting the brainstem.

➤ Red flag features that suggest central disease include reduced level of consciousness, headache, papilloedema, ataxia, dysarthria, diplopia, facial weakness or numbness, dysphagia and hemiplegia.

HISTORY[2]

➤ Time course and onset of symptoms.

➤ Pattern of symptoms:
   – Short episodes of vertigo are more likely to be peripheral than central in origin.
   – Vertigo provoked by head movement is most likely to be due to benign paroxysmal positional vertigo.

➤ Associated symptoms:
   – Influenza-like illness before the onset of vertigo is a feature of vestibular neuritis.
   – Ear pain occurs with Ramsay–Hunt syndrome, cholesteatoma and vestibular schwannoma.
   – Hearing loss and tinnitus occur more often with peripheral disorders.
   – Headache may occur with basilar migraine or posterior fossa space-occupying lesions.
   – Neck pain is a feature of vertebral artery dissection.
   – Abnormal gait or dysarthria suggests a central cause that is also affecting the cerebellum (e.g. posterior circulation ischaemia or a posterior fossa space-occupying lesion).
   – Limb weakness, dysphagia, diplopia, facial weakness or facial numbness in association with vertigo suggests brainstem pathology.

➤ Drug history.

➤ Alcohol intake.

EXAMINATION[2]

➤ Hallpike test. A sudden change in head position from upright and facing forward to lying back and facing right causes nystagmus and vertigo after a latent period of a few seconds in benign paroxysmal positional vertigo. Vertical nystagmus or lack of a latent period suggests a central cause.

➤ Eye movements and nystagmus. Nystagmus due to peripheral lesions is usually horizontal and rotatory, and is lessened by gaze fixation, whereas central nystagmus is purely horizontal, vertical or rotatory, and is not lessened by gaze fixation.

➤ Fundoscopy. Papilloedema is a sign of raised intracranial pressure.

➤ Cerebellar signs such as gait ataxia, reduced coordination and dysarthria suggest a central cause (e.g. a cerebellopontine angle tumour).

➤ Sensorineural hearing loss may occur with both central and peripheral causes of vertigo, although it more commonly occurs with peripheral causes.

➤ Limb weakness or abnormalities of cranial nerves other than VIII suggest a central cause.

INVESTIGATIONS

The following investigations may be required:

➤ Blood tests:
   – Serum magnesium.
   – Syphilis serology.
   – ANA, ENA and ANCA. These are positive in autoimmune disease or vasculitis.
   – ANNA-1 or 2. These are present in paraneoplastic brainstem encephalitis.

➤ Imaging:
   – MRI of the brain allows the diagnosis of brainstem haemorrhage or infarction, demyelination, cerebellopontine angle tumours, and other space-occupying lesions and structural abnormalities.
   – CT or MR angiogram may be diagnostic of vascular disorders such as vertebrobasilar insufficiency and subclavian steal syndrome.

➤ Specialised vestibular investigations:
   – Electronystagmography and rotational chair testing may be used to distinguish central from peripheral causes of vertigo.
   – Pneumatic otoscopy is used to detect perilymph fistula.

REFERENCES

1   Minor LB. Superior canal dehiscence syndrome. *Am J Otol*. 2000; **21(1)**: 9–19.
2   Labuguen RH. Initial evaluation of vertigo. *Am Fam Physician*. 2006; **73**: 244–51.

CHAPTER 26

Frequency of micturition

PATHOPHYSIOLOGY AND AETIOLOGY

The antidiuretic hormone (ADH)–thirst axis closely regulates serum osmolality through the release of ADH from the posterior pituitary gland and the stimulation of thirst when the serum osmolality rises above the normal range of 285–295 mOsm/l.

The kidneys, via a countercurrent exchange mechanism, maintain an increasing concentration gradient between the outer and inner medulla such that the extracellular fluid is more concentrated in the inner medulla. Urine that passes into the beginning of the collecting duct is relatively dilute and, importantly, the membrane of the collecting duct is impermeable to water. Thus, in the absence of ADH, this dilute urine is excreted, causing water loss and thus a rise in serum osmolality. In the presence of ADH, water channels (aquaporins) move into the walls of the collecting duct, allowing water to move from the tubule to the renal interstitium, resulting in more concentrated urine and the retention of water within the body.

The symptom of increased frequency of micturition arises due to either increased urine volume (polyuria) or the frequent passage of small volumes of urine.

Polyuria may result from four main mechanisms:

1. cranial diabetes insipidus (inadequate ADH production from the posterior pituitary)
2. nephrogenic diabetes insipidus (insensitivity of the renal tubule to ADH)
3. impairment of the renal medullary concentration gradient:
   - hyperglycaemia
   - diuretics
   - renal disease
4. primary polydipsia (excessive water intake, often associated with psychiatric disease).

Frequent passage of small volumes of urine may result from the following mechanisms:

1. bladder outflow obstruction
2. bladder or urethral irritation
3. bladder compression due to pelvic masses
4. neuromuscular or functional disorders that affect bladder emptying.

The causes of frequency of micturition are listed in Table 26.1, with common causes highlighted in bold type.

EMERGENCY MANAGEMENT

- Severe polyuria may cause life-threatening hypovolaemia or hypernatraemia. Provide fluid resuscitation if the patient displays clinical signs of volume depletion.
- It is important to quickly diagnose or rule out diabetic emergencies, namely diabetic ketoacidosis and hyperosmolar non-ketotic state (HONK). Check the capillary blood glucose, dip the urine for ketones, and perform an ABG analysis.
- Diabetic ketoacidosis and HONK are treated with IV fluid resuscitation, IV insulin and close monitoring of the serum potassium concentration, with replacement if it is normal or low. Note that the total body potassium level will be depleted through renal loss even if the serum level is normal, and the

Table 26.1 Causes of increased frequency of micturition

Polyuric				Non-polyuric
Nephrogenic diabetes insipidus	*Cranial diabetes insipidus*	*Impaired medullary concentration gradient*	*Primary polydipsia*	*Non-polyuric*
Electrolyte disorders ▲ **Hypercalcaemia** ▲ Hypokalaemia Drugs ▲ Lithium ▲ Amphotericin B ▲ Demeclocycline ▲ Miscellaneous Familial tubulopathies	Structural ▲ **Head injury** ▲ **Neurosurgery** ▲ Hydrocephalus Neoplasia ▲ **Pituitary adenoma** ▲ **Suprasellar tumours** ▲ Pituitary metastasis Vascular ▲ Hypoxic encephalopathy ▲ Pituitary apoplexy ▲ Arteriovenous malformation ▲ Cerebral aneurysm Inflammation ▲ Lymphocytic hypophysitis ▲ Langerhans cell histiocytosis ▲ Erdheim–Chester disease ▲ Wegener's granulomatosis ▲ Sarcoidosis ▲ Miscellaneous Infection ▲ Meningitis ▲ Encephalitis ▲ Intracranial abscess Miscellaneous ▲ Alcohol ▲ Supraventricular tachycardia[1] ▲ Gestational ▲ Familial	**Diabetes mellitus** Diabetic emergencies ▲ **Diabetic ketoacidosis** ▲ **Hyperosmolar non-ketotic state** Diuretics ▲ **Loop diuretics** ▲ **Thiazide diuretics** ▲ Osmotic diuretics ▲ Miscellaneous Chronic renal failure Acute kidney injury ▲ **Renal tract obstruction (recovery)** ▲ **Acute tubular necrosis (recovery)** ▲ Acute interstitial nephritis Tubulointerstitial disease	Psychiatric disorders ▲ Bipolar disorder ▲ Schizophrenia ▲ Anorexia nervosa Idiopathic	Prostate ▲ **Benign prostatic hyperplasia** ▲ **Prostate cancer** ▲ Prostatitis Bladder ▲ **Bacterial cystitis** ▲ Calculi ▲ Diverticulum ▲ Tumour ▲ Tuberculosis ▲ Fungal infection ▲ Schistosomiasis ▲ Interstitial cystitis ▲ Radiation cystitis ▲ Miscellaneous Urethra ▲ **Urethritis** ▲ Urethral stricture ▲ Urethral cancer ▲ Pinhole meatus ▲ Phimosis Gynaecological ▲ **Pregnancy** ▲ Uterine fibroid ▲ Ovarian cancer ▲ Ovarian cyst ▲ Uterine prolapse ▲ Miscellaneous Neuromuscular ▲ Autonomic neuropathy ▲ Myelopathy ▲ Chiari malformation ▲ Functional

concentration may fall to dangerously low levels once insulin is started, hence the importance of IV potassium replacement. The precise protocol of fluids, insulin and potassium used will depend on clinical judgement and local policies. Patients with diabetic ketoacidosis may require up to 5 litres of fluid in the first 24 hours, whereas fluid resuscitation tends to be less vigorous in the older cohort that presents with HONK.
➤ Hypernatraemia should be managed as described in Chapter 35.

HISTORY
➤ Time course of symptoms.
➤ Dysuria, urgency, strangury, hesitancy and terminal dribbling are symptoms of lower urinary tract infection, irritation or obstruction.
➤ Headache, visual field defects and other focal neurological deficits suggest hypothalamic or pituitary disease.
➤ Miscellaneous symptoms:
  – Fever suggests infection.
  – Urethral discharge occurs with urethritis.
  – Perineal pain suggests prostatitis.
➤ Past medical history.
➤ Drug history, focusing on diuretics and drugs that are known to cause nephrogenic diabetes insipidus.
➤ Family history, particularly hereditary causes of diabetes insipidus and nephropathy.
➤ Alcohol and caffeine intake.

EXAMINATION
➤ Check for signs of hypovolaemia. These include tachycardia, tachypnoea, hypotension or postural hypotension, oliguria, confusion, weak thready pulse, cool peripheries, prolonged capillary refill time, reduced skin turgor, dry mucous membranes and low JVP.
➤ Abdominal examination:
  – Suprapubic tenderness suggests cystitis or bladder outflow obstruction.
  – Palpation may reveal a distended bladder or an obstructing pelvic lesion.
  – Rectal examination may reveal prostatic enlargement or tenderness.
➤ Nervous system examination:
  – Bitemporal hemianopia suggests hypothalamic or pituitary disease impinging on the optic chiasm. Generalised CNS disease may cause a variety of other focal deficits.

INVESTIGATIONS
The following core investigations are commonly required:
➤ Capillary blood glucose.
➤ Urine dip and MC&S:
  – Nitrites and leucocytes are found with urinary tract infection.
  – Glucose is present with diabetic emergencies. The additional presence of ketones suggests diabetic ketoacidosis.
➤ Blood tests:
  – U&Es. Excessive renal water loss may cause hypernatraemia.
  – Calcium. Hypercalcaemia may cause nephrogenic diabetes insipidus.
  – Glucose. Levels are raised with diabetic emergencies.
  – PSA. Levels are raised with benign prostatic hypertrophy and prostate cancer.
➤ ABG. Diabetic ketoacidosis causes metabolic acidosis with a high anion gap.
➤ Renal tract USS. This may show evidence of urinary tract obstruction.

The following further investigations may be required:
➤ Water deprivation test (under expert supervision):
  – Water deprivation will produce an increase in serum osmolality. Failure to concentrate urine appropriately usually indicates nephrogenic or cranial diabetes insipidus.
  – A good response to exogenous vasopressin (i.e. an increase in urine osmolality) indicates cranial diabetes insipidus, whereas a poor response occurs with nephrogenic diabetes insipidus and conditions that cause an impaired medullary concentration gradient.
  – Primary polydipsia may give intermediate results, with a blunted response to both water deprivation and exogenous vasopressin, due to chronic impairment of the medullary concentration gradient.
➤ Imaging:
  – Abdominal USS or CT scan may show obstructing pelvic masses causing the frequent passage of small amounts of urine.
  – Cystoscopy may reveal tumours, calculi, diverticulae or interstitial cystitis.

- – Pituitary MRI is required to investigate cranial diabetes insipidus.
- – Spinal MRI should be performed if there is a suspicion of spinal cord pathology causing neurological disturbance of micturition.
- – Urodynamic studies may help to diagnose functional bladder disorders.

REFERENCE

1   Fujii T, Kojima S, Imanishi M *et al*. Different mechanisms of polyuria and natriuresis associated with paroxysmal supraventricular tachycardia. *Am J Cardiol*. 1991; **68**: 343–8.

CHAPTER 27

Haematuria

PATHOPHYSIOLOGY AND AETIOLOGY

Haematuria may be caused by bleeding from any part of the renal tract, precipitated by infection, inflammation, neoplasia or other miscellaneous factors. Haematuria may be visible to the naked eye (macroscopic) or detected only by microscopy or urine dip testing (microscopic). Urine may also be discoloured by haemoglobin, myoglobin, porphyrins and a variety of other substances. Such discolouration may be mistaken for haematuria, and is known as pseudohaematuria.

The causes of haematuria are listed in Table 27.1, with common causes highlighted in bold type.

EMERGENCY MANAGEMENT

➤ Severe haematuria may occasionally cause life-threatening hypovolaemia or anaemia. Provide fluid resuscitation and blood transfusion if required.
➤ Correct any bleeding disorder or coagulopathy, including reversal of anticoagulation unless this is essential.
➤ Frank haematuria may cause bladder outflow obstruction or urethral catheter occlusion due to blood clots. This should be prevented by providing bladder irrigation via a three-way catheter.

HISTORY

➤ Time course of symptoms.
➤ Timing of haematuria within the urinary stream:
  – Initial haematuria suggests urethral pathology.
  – Whole-stream haematuria occurs with upper urinary tract pathology.
  – Terminal haematuria suggests bladder pathology.
➤ Associated symptoms:
  – Loin pain occurs with ureteric colic and some renal pathologies.
  – Dysuria, frequency and urgency are symptoms of lower urinary tract disease.
  – Urethral discharge, scrotal swelling or pain, and perineal pain are features of urethritis, epididymo-orchitis and prostatitis, respectively.
➤ Sexual and menstrual history. Patients who are currently menstruating may produce urine samples contaminated with blood, thus causing false microscopic haematuria. Urethritis may be caused by sexually transmitted infections.
➤ Drug history. Rifampicin and a number of other drugs may cause discoloured urine, mimicking haematuria.

EXAMINATION

➤ General examination:
  – Fever suggests systemic infection or inflammation.
  – Skin rash or joint swelling may occur with systemic vasculitis.
  – Oedema and hypertension are features of nephritic syndrome.
➤ Abdomen:
  – Suprapubic tenderness is a feature of cystitis, whereas loin pain occurs with pyelonephritis.
  – A palpable flank mass may indicate a renal tumour.
  – Palpate carefully for an abdominal aortic aneurysm.
  – Rectal examination may reveal a tender boggy prostate (prostatitis) or a hard craggy prostatic mass (prostate cancer). Diffuse prostate enlargement may be due to benign prostatic hypertrophy or malignancy.
➤ External genitalia. Inspect for genital ulcers or other lesions.

INVESTIGATIONS

The following core investigations are commonly required:
➤ Urine dip and MC&S. Proteinuria with haematuria suggests glomerular disease, whereas the presence of red cell casts on microscopy is diagnostic of glomerulonephritis.
➤ Blood tests (FBC, U&Es, CRP and clotting screen).
➤ Renal tract USS. This may reveal renal tract calculi.
➤ Cystoscopy. This is the first-line investigation for suspected bladder malignancies.

Table 27.1 Causes of haematuria and pseudohaematuria

Infection	Neoplasia	Vascular disease	Miscellaneous	Pseudohaematuria
Local bacterial infection	Transitional-cell carcinoma	Primary glomerulopathies	Acute interstitial nephritis	Endogenous substances
➤ Cystitis	➤ Renal pelvis	➤ IgA nephropathy	Bleeding diathesis	➤ Haemoglobinuria
➤ Pyelonephritis	➤ Ureter	➤ Goodpasture's disease		➤ Myoglobinuria
➤ Tuberculosis	➤ Bladder	➤ Membranous nephropathy	Mechanical	➤ Bilirubinuria
➤ Prostatitis	➤ Urethra	➤ Mesangiocapillary	➤ Calculi	➤ Porphyria
➤ Epididymo-orchitis		glomerulonephritis	➤ Trauma	➤ Alkaptonuria
➤ Urethritis	Squamous-cell carcinoma		➤ Crystalluria	
	➤ Renal pelvis	Vasculitis	➤ Papillary necrosis	Foodstuffs
Systemic bacterial infections	➤ Ureter	➤ Wegener's granulomatosis	➤ Prostatic calculus	➤ Beetroot
➤ Leptospirosis	➤ Bladder	➤ Churg–Strauss syndrome	➤ Post-obstructive	➤ Rhubarb
➤ Legionnaire's disease	➤ Urethra	➤ Microscopic polyangiitis	➤ Foreign body	➤ Blackberry
	➤ Penis	➤ Henoch–Schönlein purpura	➤ Exercise	➤ Food colouring
Viral haemorrhagic cystitis		➤ Cryoglobulinaemia		
➤ Adenovirus	Renal tumours	➤ Renal-limited vasculitis	Familial/congenital	Drugs
➤ Cytomegalovirus	➤ Renal-cell carcinoma		➤ Thin membrane nephropathy	➤ Rifampicin
➤ BK virus	➤ Nephroblastoma	Infection	➤ Alport's syndrome	➤ Chloroquine
	➤ Lymphoma	➤ Post-streptococcal	➤ Polycystic kidney disease	➤ Metronidazole
Systemic viral infections	➤ Metastases	glomerulonephritis	➤ Medullary sponge kidney	➤ Nitrofurantoin
➤ Hantavirus		➤ Infective endocarditis	➤ Fabry's disease	➤ Desferrioxamine
➤ Yellow fever	Benign polyps	➤ HIV-associated nephropathy	➤ Nail-patella syndrome	➤ Sulphasalazine
➤ Dengue fever	➤ Renal pelvis	➤ Miscellaneous		➤ Phenytoin
➤ Viral haemorrhagic fever	➤ Bladder		Non-infectious cystitis	
	➤ Urethra	Connective tissue disease	➤ Chemotherapy	Miscellaneous
Fungal infection		➤ Systemic lupus erythematosus	➤ Radiation	➤ Utero-urethral fistula
➤ Candidiasis	Prostate cancer	➤ Rheumatoid arthritis	➤ Interstitial cystitis	➤ Menstruation
➤ Aspergillosis		➤ Mixed connective tissue disease	➤ Eosinophilic cystitis	➤ Factitious
➤ Mucormycosis			➤ Polypoid cystitis	
➤ Cryptococcosis		Small vessel disease	➤ Cystitis glandularis	
		➤ Malignant hypertension		
Helminth infection		➤ TTP/HUS	Miscellaneous renal tract lesions	
➤ Schistosomiasis		➤ Antiphospholipid syndrome	➤ Renal cyst	
➤ Paragonimiasis		➤ Systemic sclerosis	➤ Urachal cyst	
➤ Hydatid disease		➤ Pre-eclampsia	➤ Urethral caruncle	
		➤ Eclampsia	➤ Langerhans cell histiocytosis	
		➤ HELLP syndrome	➤ Inflammatory pseudotumour	
		➤ Cholesterol embolism	➤ Amyloidosis	
		➤ Sickle-cell disease		
		➤ Loin pain haematuria syndrome	Genital tract disease	
			➤ Endometriosis	
		Large vessel disease	➤ Genital ulcer	
		➤ Renal vein occlusion	➤ Benign prostatic hypertrophy	
		➤ Renal artery occlusion		
		➤ Renal artery or aortic aneurysm	Acute appendicitis[1]	
		➤ Arteriovenous malformations		
		➤ Polyarteritis nodosa		

The following further investigations may be required:
- ➤ PSA. Levels are raised in most cases of prostate cancer.
- ➤ Autoimmune profile:
  - ANA, ENA and RhF
  - anti-dsDNA (SLE)
  - ANCA (Wegener's granulomatosis, Churg–Strauss syndrome)
  - anti-GBM antibody (Goodpasture's disease)
  - anti-cardiolipin antibodies, lupus anticoagulant and anti-β2 glycoprotein I (antiphospholipid syndrome)
  - complement C3 and C4 (levels may be low with SLE)
  - cryoglobulins
  - anti-streptolysin O titre (may be raised with post-streptococcal glomerulonephritis or Henoch–Schönlein purpura).
- ➤ Imaging:
  - CXR may show airspace shadowing which suggests alveolar haemorrhage, a feature of pulmonary–renal syndromes such as Goodpasture's disease.
  - CT of the kidneys, ureters and bladder or intravenous urogram are used to diagnose urinary tract calculi or tumours.
  - Renal MR angiogram or formal angiography may be required to diagnose renal artery thrombosis.
- ➤ Renal biopsy may be required to diagnose vasculitis or connective tissue disorders involving the kidney.

REFERENCE
1   Flannigan GM, Towler JM. Appendicitis presenting with painless haematuria. *J Urol*. 1983; **129**(6): 12–48.

CHAPTER 28

Joint pain or swelling

PATHOPHYSIOLOGY AND AETIOLOGY

Joint pain or swelling may be caused by any of the following broad mechanisms:

1 systemic inflammation
2 local or systemic infection
3 degenerative or mechanical factors
4 miscellaneous causes.

The causes of joint pain or swelling are listed in Table 28.1, with common causes highlighted in bold type.

EMERGENCY MANAGEMENT

Septic arthritis is the most important diagnosis to make in a timely manner. Acute monoarthritis should be assumed to be due to septic arthritis until proved otherwise. If the patient is septic, circulatory support may be required with fluid resuscitation and possibly inotropes in a high-dependency setting. Early liaison with the orthopaedic team is essential for consideration of joint wash-out in theatre. Following blood cultures and joint aspiration for Gram stain and culture, broad-spectrum antibiotics should be commenced.

HISTORY

➤ Time course and onset of symptoms.
➤ Recent trauma or joint injury.
➤ Distribution of joint involvement:
  – Establish whether it is monoarthritis or polyarthritis. Septic arthritis and crystal arthropathies classically present with acute monoarthritis, whereas connective tissue diseases cause polyarthritis.
  – Large or small joint involvement.
  – Symmetrical or asymmetrical.
  – Migratory or fixed.
➤ Associated symptoms:
  – Significant morning stiffness suggests an inflammatory arthritis such as rheumatoid arthritis.
  – Fever and rigors occur with septic arthritis.
  – Skin rash may occur with connective tissue disease, vasculitis and some systemic infections such as disseminated gonococcaemia.
  – Sore throat may occur in association with post-streptococcal arthritis, gonococcal arthritis and rheumatic fever.
  – Genital discharge or ulceration suggests reactive arthritis, gonococcal arthritis, syphilis or Behçet's disease.
  – Diarrhoea suggests an enteropathic arthritis such as inflammatory bowel disease-related arthritis.
  – Mouth ulcers occur with Behçet's disease and Crohn's disease.
  – Dry eyes and mouth are a feature of Sjögren's syndrome.
  – Ocular pain or erythema may occur with sarcoidosis, rheumatoid arthritis or the spondyloarthritides.
➤ Social history:
  – Foreign travel.
  – Sexual history. Risky sexual behaviour suggests the possibility of gonococcal arthritis, secondary syphilis or reactive arthritis.

EXAMINATION

➤ General examination:
  – Check the vital signs (pulse, blood pressure, respiratory rate and temperature).
  – Skin rash may be associated with psoriasis, vasculitis, SLE and disseminated infection, particularly secondary syphilis or gonococcaemia.
  – Check for features of systemic sclerosis, including tight skin, microstomia, sclerodactyly, telangiectasias, subcutaneous calcification and Raynaud's phenomenon.
  – Characteristic subcutaneous tophi may be seen with gout.
➤ Joint examination:
  – Joint swelling, warmth or erythema suggests active inflammation or infection.

Table 28.1 Causes of joint pain or swelling

Inflammation	*Infection*	*Mechanical*	*Miscellaneous*
Collagen vascular disease	Septic arthritis	Degenerative disease	Crystal arthropathies
▲ Rheumatoid arthritis	▲ Gonococcal	▲ Osteoarthritis	▲ Gout
▲ Systemic lupus erythematosus	▲ Non-gonococcal	▲ Adhesive capsulitis	▲ Pseudogout
▲ Systemic sclerosis	Tuberculous arthritis	▲ Osteonecrosis	▲ Chronic pyrophosphate arthropathy
▲ Sjögren's syndrome		▲ Regional migratory osteoporosis[4]	▲ Acute calcific periarthritis
▲ Mixed connective tissue disease	Aseptic bacterial arthritis		▲ Apatite-associated destructive arthritis
▲ Dermatomyositis	▲ Lyme disease	Trauma	▲ Miscellaneous
▲ Polymyositis	▲ Brucellosis	▲ Fracture	
▲ Polymyalgia rheumatica	▲ Rat-bite fever	▲ Haemarthrosis	Endocrine, toxic and metabolic
▲ Adult Still's disease	▲ Relapsing fever	▲ Ligament rupture	▲ Osteomalacia
▲ Relapsing polychondritis	▲ Syphilis	▲ Tendon rupture	▲ Renal osteodystrophy
▲ RS3PE syndrome	▲ Yaws	▲ Rotator cuff tear	▲ Hyperparathyroidism
	▲ Leprosy	▲ Ruptured Baker's cyst	▲ Amyloidosis
Spondyloarthritides	▲ Miscellaneous	▲ Foreign body	▲ Haemochromatosis
▲ Ankylosing spondylitis			▲ Wilson's disease
▲ Reactive arthritis	Viral infection	Overuse injury	▲ Ochronosis
▲ Psoriatic arthritis	▲ Parvovirus B19	▲ Tendinitis	▲ Sitosterolaemia
▲ IBD-related arthritis	▲ Hepatitis A, B and C	▲ Bursitis	▲ Hyperlipidaemia
▲ Undifferentiated spondyloarthropathy	▲ Adenovirus	▲ Chondromalacia	▲ Hypothyroidism
▲ SAPHO syndrome	▲ Enterovirus	▲ Osteochondritis dissecans	▲ Acromegaly
	▲ Influenza	▲ Plica syndrome	▲ Adrenal insufficiency
Vasculitis	▲ Epstein–Barr virus	▲ Distal clavicle osteolysis	▲ Scurvy
▲ Wegener's granulomatosis	▲ Rubella		▲ Kashin–Beck disease
▲ Churg–Strauss syndrome	▲ Mumps		▲ Drugs and toxins
▲ Microscopic polyangiitis	▲ HIV		
▲ Polyarteritis nodosa	▲ HTLV-1		Vascular
▲ Cryoglobulinaemia	▲ West Nile virus		▲ Sickle-cell crisis
▲ Henoch–Schönlein purpura	▲ Dengue fever		▲ Decompression sickness
▲ Kawasaki disease	▲ Chikurgunya		▲ TTP/HUS
▲ Behçet's disease	▲ Miscellaneous		
▲ Takayasu arteritis			Neoplasia
	Miscellaneous		▲ Multiple myeloma
Infection-related	▲ Fungi		▲ Bone metastases
▲ Rheumatic fever	▲ Protozoa		▲ Primary bone tumours
▲ Post-streptococcal arthritis	▲ Helminths		▲ Synovial tumours
▲ Endocarditis			▲ Acute leukaemia
			▲ Lymphoma
Familial periodic fever			
▲ Familial Mediterranean fever			
▲ Muckle–Wells syndrome			
▲ Familial cold urticaria			
▲ TRAPS			
▲ HIDS			
▲ CINCA syndrome			
▲ PAPA syndrome			
▲ Blau syndrome			
Gastrointestinal conditions			
▲ Coeliac disease			
▲ Microscopic colitis			
▲ Intestinal bypass surgery			
▲ Whipple's disease			
Dermatological conditions			
▲ Acne arthralgia			
▲ Pyoderma gangrenosum			
▲ Erythema multiforme			
▲ Stevens–Johnson syndrome			
▲ Toxic epidermal necrolysis			
▲ Hypocomplementaemic urticarial vasculitis			
▲ Sweet's syndrome			
▲ Schnitzler syndrome			
▲ Multicentric reticulohistiocytosis[1]			
▲ Fibroblastic rheumatism[1]			
▲ Erythema nodosum			
▲ Pancreatic panniculitis[2]			
▲ Weber–Christian disease			
▲ Eosinophilia–myalgia syndrome			
▲ Eosinophilic fasciitis			
Miscellaneous			
▲ Sarcoidosis			
▲ Serum sickness			
▲ Acute interstitial nephritis			
▲ Atrial myxoma			
▲ Hypereosinophilic syndrome			
▲ AILD			
▲ Dressler's syndrome			

continued

Table 28.1 Causes of joint pain or swelling – *continued*

Inflammation	Infection	Mechanical	Miscellaneous
➤ Carcinomatous polyarthritis[3] ➤ Intermittent hydrarthrosis ➤ Macrophagic myofasciitis ➤ Human adjuvant disease			*Proliferative conditions* ➤ Pigmented villonodular synovitis ➤ Synovial osteochondromatosis ➤ Hypertrophic pulmonary osteoarthropathy *Neuropathic* ➤ Spinal cord compression ➤ Syringomyelia ➤ Acute brachial plexus neuritis ➤ Thoracic outlet obstruction ➤ Compression radiculopathy ➤ Peripheral nerve compression ➤ Reflex sympathetic dystrophy ➤ Charcot's arthropathy *Referred shoulder pain* ➤ Diaphragmatic irritation ➤ Cervical spine pathology ➤ Cardiac ischaemia ➤ Pericarditis

- Swan-neck, Boutonnière and Z-thumb deformities, and ulnar deviation at the metacarpophalyngeal joints, are features of rheumatoid arthritis.
- Heberden's and Bouchard's nodes occur with osteoarthritis.
- Examine active and passive movements. Patients with septic arthritis will often not allow any movement of the joint due to the pain that this causes, but this is **not** an invariable feature. Joint crepitus is a feature of osteoarthritis.

INVESTIGATIONS

The following core investigations are commonly required:

➤ Blood tests:
  - FBC may reveal anaemia of chronic disease, or neutrophilia, suggesting bacterial infection.
  - ESR and CRP are raised with infection or inflammation.
  - U&Es may be deranged with severe sepsis in association with joint infection.
  - Calcium levels are raised with myeloma, bone metastases and primary bone tumours, but are low in osteomalacia.
  - ALP levels are raised with malignant bone infiltration and osteomalacia.
  - Uric acid levels may be raised with gout.
  - ANA and RhF may be positive with connective tissue disease and rheumatoid arthritis, respectively.
  - Blood culture should be performed if there are features of sepsis.
➤ Joint aspirate microscopy and culture:
  - Turbid aspirate with leucocytes suggests septic arthritis. Microscopy may reveal bacteria with Gram stain, or acid-fast bacilli with Ziehl–Neelsen stain.
  - Crystals are seen with gout, pseudogout and other crystal arthropathies.
  - Culture.
➤ Urine dip should be performed, as haematuria may occur with systemic vasculitis or infective endocarditis.
➤ ECG is mandatory in cases of shoulder pain, as myocardial ischaemia may cause pain that radiates to the arm or shoulder.
➤ Plain radiograph of the affected joint(s) may show osteophytes, bone cysts, subchondral sclerosis and joint space narrowing, all of which are features of osteoarthritis. Chondrocalcinosis may be seen with pseudogout. Erosions are characteristic of rheumatoid arthritis. Subluxations and other deformities may be visualised.

The following further investigations may be required:

➤ Biochemistry and immunology:
  - Serum electrophoresis, serum free light chains and urinary Bence Jones protein are used to diagnose multiple myeloma.
  - Autoimmune screen includes ANA, anti-dsDNA (SLE), RhF (rheumatoid arthritis), ANCA (Churg–Strauss syndrome, Wegener's granulomatosis), anti-Ro and anti-La (Sjögren's syndrome), anti-RNP (mixed connective tissue disease) and cryoglobulins.
  - Tissue transglutaminase, anti-endomysial and antigliadin antibodies are positive in coeliac disease.
  - HLA-B27 testing may be helpful in the diagnosis of the spondyloarthritides.
  - Serum ACE levels are raised with sarcoidosis.
  - Vitamin D levels are low in osteomalacia.
  - Ferritin is raised with haemochromatosis and adult Still's disease.
➤ Microbiology:
  - Viral serology or PCR for parvovirus B19, enterovirus, EBV, CMV, HSV, VZV, hepatitis A, B or C, HIV, alphavirus and flavivirus.
  - Lyme or *Brucella* serology.
  - TPHA and VDRL are positive with syphilis and yaws.
  - Duodenal biopsy. PAS-positive macrophages and positive *Tropheryma whipplei* PCR are diagnostic of Whipple's disease.
➤ Imaging:
  - Joint MRI provides more detail of soft tissue pathology.
  - Skeletal survey may show evidence of multiple myeloma, metastatic malignancy or primary bone tumours.

REFERENCES

1   Pedersen JK, Poulsen T, Hørslev-Petersen K. Fibroblastic rheumatism: a Scandinavian case report. *Ann Rheum Dis*. 2005; 64: 156–7.
2   Watts RA, Kelly S, Hacking JC *et al*. Fat necrosis. An unusual cause of polyarthritis. *J Rheumatol*. 1993; 20(8): 1432–5.
3   Zupancic M, Annamalai A, Brenneman J *et al*. Migratory polyarthritis as a paraneoplastic syndrome. *J Gen Intern Med*. 2008; 23(12): 2136–9.
4   Cahir JG, Toms AP. Regional migratory osteoporosis. *Eur J Radiol*. 2008; 67(1): 2–10.

CHAPTER 29

Back pain

PATHOPHYSIOLOGY AND AETIOLOGY

Back pain may be caused by disease affecting a wide variety of anatomical structures covering the full spectrum of pathological processes, including degeneration, structural abnormalities, infection, inflammation, neoplasia, ischaemia and haemorrhage. As such the differential diagnosis is wide, and although most cases seen in primary care are caused by relatively benign pathology, such as osteoarthritis, more serious causes must always be considered, especially in the cohort of patients who present acutely to hospital.

Back pain is most conveniently classified according to the structure or organ that is the source of pain, as follows:

1   spine and nervous system:
    a   spine
    b   spinal cord
    c   spinal nerve roots
2   retroperitoneal structures:
    a   renal tract
    b   genital tract
    c   abdominal aorta
    d   pancreas
    e   gastrointestinal tract
    f   miscellaneous
3   thoracic structures:
    a   thoracic aorta
    b   heart
    c   pleura
    d   oesophagus
4   paraspinal muscles
5   diaphragm (causing referred shoulder tip pain)
6   miscellaneous.

The differential diagnosis of back pain is shown in Table 29.1, with common causes highlighted in bold type.

EMERGENCY MANAGEMENT

➤ There are a number of red flag diagnoses that should not be missed, as timely treatment may prevent permanent neurological disability, or even death. They include the following:
   – cauda equina syndrome
   – spinal cord compression
   – spinal infection or malignant infiltration
   – leaking abdominal aortic aneurysm
   – aortic dissection.
➤ Specific treatment will depend on the underlying cause. For example, cauda equina syndrome, spinal cord compression, leaking abdominal aortic aneurysm and type A aortic dissection require urgent surgical intervention to prevent neurological damage or death. Infection of the spine requires prolonged courses of antimicrobial or antituberculous chemotherapy as appropriate. Spinal surgery may be required to stabilise the vertebral column.

HISTORY

➤ A history of recent trauma or heavy lifting suggests a mechanical cause of the pain, such as a prolapsed intervertebral disc. Neurosurgical emergencies such as spinal cord compression and cauda equina syndrome should be excluded.
➤ Time course and onset:
   – Sudden onset implies a vascular or mechanical event (e.g. ruptured aortic aneurysm, aortic dissection or prolapsed intervertebral disc).
   – Subacute onset suggests infection, inflammation or malignancy.
   – Chronic pain occurs with degenerative conditions.

Table 29.1 Causes of back pain[1]

Spinal and neurological

Neurosurgical emergencies
- Cauda equina syndrome
- Spinal cord compression

Degenerative/mechanical
- Muscle strain
- Osteoarthritis
- Vertebral or rib fracture
- Spondylolisthesis
- Intervertebral disc prolapse
- Spinal stenosis
- Vertebral osteochondritis
- Charcot arthropathy

Neoplasia
- Vertebral metastases
- Multiple myeloma
- Primary bone tumour
- Langerhans cell histiocytosis
- Leukaemia
- Mastocytosis
- Lymphoma
- Castleman's disease
- Spinal cord tumour
- Haemangioma
- Lipoma
- Malignant peripheral nerve sheath tumour

Endocrine and metabolic
- Osteomalacia
- Renal osteodystrophy
- Hyperparathyroidism
- Paget's disease
- Acromegaly
- Haemochromatosis
- Ochronosis
- Gout
- Miscellaneous

Inflammatory arthritis
- Polymyalgia rheumatica
- Ankylosing spondylitis
- Psoriatic arthritis
- Reactive arthritis
- Enteropathic arthritis
- Undifferentiated spondyloarthropathy
- SAPHO syndrome
- Acne arthralgia
- Familial Mediterranean fever

Vascular
- Subarachnoid haemorrhage
- Subdura haematoma
- Epidural haematoma
- Spinal cord haemorrhage
- Spinal cord infarction
- Vascular malformation
- Cavernous angioma
- Decompression sickness
- Sickle-cell crisis

Structural abnormalities
- Syringomyelia
- Spinal dysraphism
- Tarlov cyst

Miscellaneous
- Shingles
- Post-herpetic neuralgia
- Diabetic radiculopathy
- Guillain-Barré syndrome
- Transverse myelitis
- Vertebral sarcoidosis
- Chronic recurrent multifocal osteomyelitis
- Multicentric reticulohistiocytosis
- Extramedullary haemopoiesis
- Schnitzler syndrome

Retroperitoneal and pelvic structures

Vascular
- Abdominal aortic aneurysm
- Retroperitoneal haemorrhage

Renal
- Ureteric colic
- Renal calculi
- Pyelonephritis
- Renal abscess
- Perinephric abscess
- Renal tuberculosis
- Renal infarction
- Renal malignancy
- Hydronephrosis
- Renal cyst haemorrhage
- Glomerulonephritis
- Acute interstitial nephritis
- Loin pain haematuria syndrome

Pancreatic
- Acute pancreatitis
- Chronic pancreatitis
- Pancreatic cancer

Gastrointestinal
- Peptic ulcer
- Appendicitis
- Diverticulitis
- Rectal cancer

Gynaecological
- Ectopic pregnancy
- Pelvic inflammatory disease
- Ovarian torsion
- Ovarian cancer
- Mumps oophoritis
- Endometriosis

Thoracic structures

Thoracic aorta
- Aortic dissection
- Intramural aortic haematoma
- Penetrating aortic ulcer
- Thoracic aortic aneurysm

Cardiac ischaemia
- Myocardial infarction
- Angina pectoris

Pleural
- Pulmonary embolism
- Pneumothorax
- Pneumonia
- Empyema
- Haemothorax
- Lung cancer
- Malignant mesothelioma
- Miscellaneous

Oesophageal
- Spasm
- Malignancy
- Rupture

Miscellaneous

Referred pain from diaphragmatic irritation
- Subphrenic abscess
- Hepatic abscess
- Cholecystitis
- Peritonitis
- Intra-abdominal haemorrhage

Systemic viral infection
- Influenza
- Dengue fever
- Yellow fever
- Chikungunya
- West Nile virus
- Miscellaneous

Systemic bacterial infection
- Leptospirosis
- Relapsing fever
- Trench fever
- Rickettsiosis

Toxic and metabolic
- Acute porphyria
- Acute intravascular haemolysis[2]
- Opioid withdrawal

Chronic pain syndromes
- Coccydynia
- Fibromyalgia

continued

Table 29.1 Causes of back pain[1] – *continued*

Spinal and neurological	Retroperitoneal and pelvic structures	Thoracic structures	Miscellaneous
Infection	Prostatitic and testicular		
➤ **Bacterial osteomyelitis**	➤ Prostatitis		
➤ **Pyogenic discitis**	➤ Prostate cancer		
➤ Pyogenic sacroiliitis	➤ Testicular cancer		
➤ Epidural abscess			
➤ Subdural empyema	Miscellaneous retroperitoneal		
➤ Intramedullary abscess	conditions		
➤ Tuberculosis	➤ Abscess		
➤ Fungal osteomyelitis	➤ Haematoma		
➤ Echinococcal osteomyelitis	➤ Tumour		
➤ Lyme disease	➤ Fibrosis		
➤ Syphilis			
➤ Yaws			
➤ Whipple's disease			

➤ Pattern of symptoms:
  – Pain that is worse at the end of the day occurs with degenerative and mechanical conditions.
  – Pain that is worse in the morning, or prolonged morning stiffness, suggests an inflammatory arthritis.
  – Unremitting pain that keeps the patient awake at night is characteristic of vertebral malignancy or infection.
➤ Location of pain and radiation:
  – Flank pain suggests renal tract or ovarian pathology. Radiation to the groin is characteristic of ureteric colic.
  – Thoracic pain and lumbosacral pain may be caused by pathology affecting thoracic and retroperitoneal structures, respectively.
  – Pain arising from the spine or spinal cord is usually localised to the anatomical level of the pathological process.
  – Shoulder tip pain is caused by subdiaphragmatic pathology causing referred pain.
  – Radiation down the back of the thigh (sciatica) suggests nerve root compression. Unilateral or bilateral sciatica may be a feature of cauda equina syndrome.
➤ Character and severity of pain:
  – Severe colicky pain occurs with ureteric colic. The patient is characteristically unable to lie still due to the severity of the pain.
  – Sharp, stabbing or shooting pain is characteristic of nerve root impingement.
➤ Exacerbating and relieving factors:
  – Pain due to mechanical injury or degeneration is particularly aggravated by back movement.
  – Pain arising from pleural irritation is exacerbated by inspiration or coughing.
  – The pain of pancreatitis may be relieved by leaning forward.
➤ Associated symptoms:
  – Fever, weight loss or night sweats may occur with infection, inflammation or malignancy.
  – Weakness, gait disturbance or altered sensation suggests spinal cord or nerve root impingement.
  – Urinary or faecal incontinence, urinary retention, constipation or perineal anaesthesia in a 'saddle' distribution are symptoms of cauda equina syndrome, and urgent spinal imaging is mandatory.
  – Haematuria occurs with renal tract calculi, infection or malignancy.
  – Diarrhoea or genital discharge raises the possibility of reactive arthritis.
  – Abnormal vaginal discharge or bleeding suggests gynaecological pathology.

EXAMINATION
➤ Check the vital signs. Tachycardia or hypotension in association with back pain may indicate an aortic dissection or leaking abdominal aortic aneurysm.
➤ Inspect the spine for scoliosis or kyphosis.
➤ Focal tenderness may suggest the site of pathology. For example, tenderness directly over the spine may be due to bony injury, osteomyelitis or malignant infiltration, whereas flank tenderness may be due to renal pathology.
➤ Neurological system:
  – Spastic paraplegia or quadriplegia with brisk reflexes and up-going plantar responses is consistent with spinal cord damage. An accompanying sensory level may be present.
  – Flaccid paralysis with sensory loss may occur with nerve root impingement (including cauda equina syndrome) or Guillain–Barré syndrome.
  – Anal tone and perianal sensation may be lost with cauda equina syndrome.
  – Perform the straight leg raise test. Sciatica on either side, particularly in the contralateral leg, suggests lumbosacral root impingement and possibly cauda equina syndrome.
➤ Check carefully for a pulsatile abdominal mass that may represent an abdominal aortic aneurysm.
➤ Delayed or absent pulses, or a blood pressure difference between the two arms, suggests aortic dissection.
➤ Percussion and auscultation of the chest may reveal evidence of pneumonia or pleural effusion that is causing pleuritic pain.

INVESTIGATIONS
The following core investigations are commonly required:
➤ Blood tests:
  – FBC, ESR and CRP may provide evidence of infection.
  – Calcium and phosphate levels are both low with osteomalacia.
  – LFTs and amylase may be deranged with hepatobiliary disease and pancreatitis, respectively.
➤ Urine dip and MC&S. Haematuria occurs with renal tract calculi, infection or malignancy, whereas leucocytes and nitrites suggest infection.
➤ Imaging:
  – CXR may show pulmonary or pleural pathology causing pleuritic back pain.

- Thoracic/lumbar spine X-ray may show evidence of malignant infiltration, osteomyelitis, fracture, spondylolisthesis or degenerative change. Fused vertebrae or sacroiliitis suggest ankylosing spondylitis.
➤ ECG. Myocardial ischaemia may occasionally cause thoracic back pain, or more commonly chest pain radiating to the back.

The following further investigations may be required:
➤ Serum electrophoresis, serum free light chains and urinary Bence Jones protein. These tests should be performed if multiple myeloma is suspected.
➤ HLA-B27 testing may aid the diagnosis of ankylosing spondylitis and other spondyloarthritides.
➤ Imaging:
- MRI of the spine is necessary for the diagnosis of spinal cord compression and cauda equina syndrome, and provides excellent visualisation of structural abnormalities, malignant infiltration and vertebral infection.
- CT of the chest with contrast is required for the diagnosis of aortic dissection or pulmonary embolism.
- Abdominal CT or USS may visualise an abdominal aortic aneurysm, abdominal collection, ectopic pregnancy or renal tract calculus.
- Intravenous urogram is used to diagnose renal tract calculi.
- OGD may allow visualisation of a posterior duodenal ulcer that is causing back pain.

REFERENCES
1   Borenstein DG, Wiesel SW, Boden SD. *Low Back and Neck Pain*. 3rd ed. Philadelphia, PA: Saunders; 2004.
2   Rother RP, Bell L, Hillmen P *et al*. The clinical sequelae of intravascular haemolysis and extracellular plasma haemoglobin. *JAMA*. 2005; **293**: 1653–62.

CHAPTER 30

Pyrexia of unknown origin

PATHOPHYSIOLOGY AND AETIOLOGY

Pyrexia is defined as a core temperature above 38°C. Core body temperature is closely regulated by the hypothalamus such that under normal circumstances it remains within the range 36.5–37.5°C. A wide range of infectious, inflammatory, neoplastic and miscellaneous conditions may result in a raised core temperature through the release of cytokines that act to up-regulate the hypothalamic temperature set point. The classical form of pyrexia of unknown origin (PUO), discussed in this chapter, may be most simply defined as pyrexia that lasts for longer than three weeks and remains undiagnosed following initial clinical assessment and investigations, comprising three days of inpatient investigation or two physician visits.[1] This definition excludes patients who are hospitalised at the time of onset of fever, and those with neutropenia or HIV infection, as a distinctly different approach to investigation and treatment is required in these cases. Table 30.1 lists the causes of classical pyrexia of unknown origin, with common causes highlighted in bold type.

EMERGENCY MANAGEMENT

In general, efforts should be made to reach a diagnosis before initiating empirical treatment that may mask or even worsen the underlying condition. However, therapeutic trials of corticosteroids, antibiotics or anti-tuberculous chemotherapy may be justified in patients who are extremely unwell.

HISTORY

➤ Time course of fever.
➤ A complete systemic review covering all systems should be performed. Particular note should be taken of the following:
  – Weight loss suggests serious underlying disease such as malignancy or chronic infection.
  – Rigors suggest infection.
  – Night sweats are characteristic of lymphoma and tuberculosis.
  – Pruritus commonly occurs with lymphoma.
  – Bone or joint pain suggests osteomyelitis or connective tissue disease.
  – Skin rash may be caused by vasculitis, connective tissue disease or systemic infection.
  – Abdominal pain suggests intra-abdominal abscess or malignancy.
  – Genital lesions or discharge may occur with genitourinary tract infections.
➤ Drug history. Drug fevers are a possible cause of PUO.
➤ Family history. Note any history of familial periodic fever.
➤ Social history:
  – travel and immunisation history
  – sexual history
  – intravenous drug abuse and tattoos
  – occupation
  – contact with animals.

EXAMINATION

➤ General examination:
  – Skin rash suggests vasculitis, connective tissue disease or systemic infection.
  – Splinter haemorrhages, Osler nodes, Janeway lesions and clubbing are signs of infective endocarditis visible on the hands. Clubbing also occurs with inflammatory bowel disease and lung cancer.
  – Goitre may occur with hyperthyroidism or subacute thyroiditis.
  – Jaundice is a feature of hepatobiliary or pancreatic disease, as well as haemolysis.
  – Lymphadenopathy occurs with lymphoma and other lymphoproliferative disorders, leukaemia, metastatic malignancy and some systemic infections.
➤ Systems examination:
  – Cardiac murmurs are audible in many cases of infective endocarditis.
  – Abdominal tenderness or mass may be due to abscess, malignancy, inflammatory bowel disease, diverticulitis or colitis.
  – Rectal examination may reveal colorectal or prostate cancer. Localised tenderness may be caused by prostatitis or perirectal abscess.

Table 30.1 Causes of pyrexia of unknown origin[1, 2]

Infection	Inflammation	Neoplasia	Miscellaneous

Infection

Bacterial abscess
➤ Subphrenic
➤ Hepatic or splenic
➤ Diverticular or perirectal
➤ Psoas
➤ Pelvic
➤ Renal or perinephric
➤ Prostatic
➤ Miscellaneous

Localised bacterial infection
➤ Infective endocarditis
➤ Osteomyelitis
➤ Urinary tract infection
➤ Prostatitis
➤ Biliary sepsis
➤ Actinomycosis

Systemic viral infection
➤ HIV seroconversion
➤ Cytomegalovirus
➤ Infectious mononucleosis
➤ Miscellaneous

Systemic bacterial infection
➤ Tuberculosis
➤ Brucellosis
➤ Lyme disease
➤ Syphilis
➤ Leptospirosis
➤ Rat bite fever
➤ Relapsing fever
➤ Ehrlichiosis
➤ Rickettsiosis
➤ Scrub typhus
➤ Q fever
➤ Bartonellosis
➤ Melioidosis
➤ Tularaemia
➤ Typhoid fever

Inflammation

Connective tissue disease
➤ Polymyalgia rheumatica
➤ Adult Still's disease
➤ Rheumatoid arthritis
➤ Systemic lupus erythematosus
➤ Mixed connective tissue disease
➤ Polymyositis
➤ Sjögren's syndrome
➤ Relapsing polychondritis
➤ Reactive arthritis
➤ Ankylosing spondylitis

Vasculitis
➤ Giant-cell arteritis
➤ Takayasu arteritis
➤ Polyarteritis nodosa
➤ Microscopic polyangiitis
➤ Wegener's granulomatosis
➤ Churg–Strauss syndrome
➤ Goodpasture's disease
➤ Cryoglobulinaemia
➤ Behçet's disease
➤ Kawasaki disease

Familial periodic fevers
➤ Familial Mediterranean fever
➤ Muckle–Wells syndrome
➤ Familial cold urticaria
➤ HIDS
➤ TRAPS

Hepatobiliary and pancreatic
➤ Autoimmune hepatitis
➤ Alcoholic hepatitis
➤ Acalculous cholecystitis
➤ Primary sclerosing cholangitis
➤ Primary biliary cirrhosis
➤ Pancreatitis

Gastrointestinal
➤ Inflammatory bowel disease

Neoplasia

Haematological
➤ Lymphoma
➤ Leukaemia
➤ Multiple myeloma
➤ Lymphomatoid granulomatosis
➤ Castleman's disease
➤ Angioimmunoblastic lymphadenopathy with dysproteinaemia
➤ Langerhans cell histiocytosis
➤ Haemophagocytic lymphohistiocytosis
➤ Rosai–Dorfman disease
➤ Malignant histiocytosis
➤ Mastocytosis

Non-haematological
➤ Renal-cell carcinoma
➤ Hepatocellular carcinoma
➤ Hepatic metastases
➤ Oesophageal
➤ Gastric
➤ Colorectal
➤ Pancreatic
➤ Biliary tract
➤ Ovarian
➤ Cervical
➤ Uterine
➤ Breast
➤ Atrial myxoma
➤ Sarcoma
➤ Mesothelioma
➤ Nasopharyngeal carcinoma
➤ Miscellaneous

Miscellaneous

Factitious fever

Drugs and toxins
➤ Drug fevers
➤ Metal/polymer fume fever
➤ Serum sickness

Granulomatous and fibrotic conditions
➤ Sarcoidosis
➤ Granulomatous hepatitis
➤ Retroperitoneal fibrosis[3]
➤ Sclerosing mesenteritis[4]
➤ IgG4-associated multifocal systemic fibrosis[5]

Haematological
➤ Pernicious anaemia
➤ Cyclical neutropenia
➤ Paroxysmal nocturnal haemoglobinuria
➤ Paroxysmal cold haemoglobinuria
➤ Thrombotic thrombocytopaenic purpura

Endocrine
➤ Hyperthyroidism
➤ Adrenal insufficiency
➤ Phaeochromocytoma

Vascular
➤ Aortic dissection
➤ Intramural aortic haematoma[6]
➤ Intra-abdominal haematoma
➤ Aortoenteric fistula[7]
➤ Pulmonary embolism
➤ Deep vein thrombosis
➤ Thrombophlebitis

Hereditary
➤ Fabry's disease
➤ Gaucher's disease

Infection

► Chronic salmonellosis
► Mycoplasma pneumonia
► Psittacosis
► Lymphogranuloma venereum
► Chronic meningococcaemia
► Disseminated gonococcaemia

Fungal infection
► Histoplasmosis
► Coccidioidomycosis
► Blastomycosis

Protozoan or helminth infection
► **Malaria**
► Babesiosis
► Visceral leishmaniasis
► African trypanosomiasis
► Toxoplasmosis
► Amoebic liver abscess
► Hydatid cyst

Inflammation

► Diverticulitis
► Whipple's disease

Cardiovascular
► Pericarditis
► Post-pericardiotomy syndrome
► Dressler's syndrome
► Rheumatic fever
► Aortitis

Miscellaneous
► Sinusitis
► Hypersensitivity pneumonitis
► Subacute thyroiditis
► Malignant meningitis
► Vogt-Koyanagi-Harada syndrome
► Kikuchi disease
► Malakoplakia

Neoplasia

Miscellaneous

Temperature dysregulation
► Hypothalamic tumour
► Hypothalamic stroke
► Diencephalic epilepsy
► Traumatic brain injury

– Mouth ulcers are a feature of Behçet's disease and Crohn's disease.
– Genital discharge or ulcer suggests a possible genitourinary focus of infection. Behçet's disease is a further cause of genital ulceration.
– Examine the breasts for signs of breast cancer.
– Focal neurological deficits may be due to intracranial abscess, encephalitis or meningitis.
– Fundoscopy may reveal the characteristic Roth spots of infective endocarditis.

INVESTIGATIONS

Investigation should be tailored to the findings elicited by careful clinical assessment, as a blanket approach is both wasteful of resources and likely to lead to misleading false-positive results. The following core investigations are commonly required:

➤ Blood tests:
– ESR and CRP are raised with infection or inflammation.
– FBC may reveal neutrophilia (bacterial infection), eosinophilia (parasitic infection, hypereosinophilic syndrome) or anaemia (chronic infection or inflammation, malignancy).
– LFTs may be deranged with granulomatous hepatitis or other hepatobiliary disease.
– TFTs. Hyperthyroidism may cause pyrexia.
– LDH is raised with lymphoma, lymphoproliferative disorders and haemolysis.
– Serum electrophoresis, serum free light chains and urinary Bence Jones protein are diagnostic investigations for multiple myeloma.
– Autoimmune and vasculitis screen includes ANA, anti-dsDNA (SLE), RhF (rheumatoid arthritis), ANCA (Churg–Strauss syndrome, Wegener's granulomatosis), anti-Ro and anti-La (Sjögren's syndrome), anti-Jo-1 (polymyositis, dermatomyositis), anti-RNP (mixed connective tissue disease), anti-GBM (Goodpasture's syndrome), anti-SMA and anti-LKM-1 (autoimmune hepatitis), AMA (primary biliary cirrhosis) and cryoglobulins.

➤ Urinalysis. Leucocytes or nitrites indicate urinary tract infection, whereas haematuria may occur with urinary tract malignancy or infection, systemic vasculitis or infective endocarditis.

➤ Microbiology:
– blood culture
– urine MC&S
– early-morning urine sample for acid-fast bacilli
– sputum MC&S, including Ziehl–Neelsen stain and mycobacterial culture
– CSF MC&S
– stool MC&S and *Clostridium difficile* toxin
– viral serology with or without PCR for HIV, CMV, EBV, and hepatitis A, B and C
– serology with or without PCR for syphilis, *Brucella*, Lyme disease, rickettsia, Q-fever, *Bartonella* or *Chlamydia*
– anti-streptolysin O titre is raised in streptococcal infection, suggesting the possibility of rheumatic fever in the appropriate clinical context
– Mantoux test is positive with tuberculosis or previous BCG immunisation.

➤ Imaging:
– CXR with or without CT of the chest may reveal a number of pathologies, including tuberculosis, lung abscess or lung cancer.
– USS or CT of the abdomen and pelvis may visualise an abscess or malignancy.

The following further investigations may be required:

➤ Biochemistry:
– Vitamin B_{12} levels are low in pernicious anaemia.
– Twenty-four-hour urinary catecholamines and VMA are used to diagnose phaeochromocytoma.
– Amylase activity is raised with pancreatitis.
– Serum ACE activity is raised with sarcoidosis.
– The short tetracosactide test is used to diagnose adrenal insufficiency.
– Tumour markers (PSA, CEA, CA 19-9 and CA-125).

➤ Haematology:
– D-dimer levels are raised with pulmonary embolism or deep vein thrombosis.
– Thick and thin films may be required to diagnose malaria, babesiosis, bartonellosis or trypanosomiasis.
– Blood film may reveal schistocytes in cases of intravascular haemolysis.
– Reticulocyte count is raised with haemolysis.
– A haemoglobinopathy screen should be performed if there is evidence of haemolysis.
– Ham's test is positive with paroxysmal nocturnal haemoglobinuria.
– Direct Coomb's test is positive in immune haemolytic anaemias.

➤ Histology and cytology:
– Liver biopsy may reveal granulomatous hepatitis, autoimmune hepatitis, primary biliary cirrhosis or primary sclerosing cholangitis.

- – Bone-marrow biopsy and culture may reveal tuberculosis, fungal infection, leukaemia, multiple myeloma or haemophagocytic lymphohistiocytosis.
- – Lymph node biopsy may be diagnostic of lymphoma, lymphoproliferative disorders, metastatic malignancy, tuberculosis or fungal infection.
- – Temporal artery biopsy is used to diagnose giant-cell arteritis.
- – Biopsy of mass lesions may allow diagnosis of malignancy or fibrosing, inflammatory or infective masses.
- – CSF cytology may reveal malignant meningitis.
- ➤ Imaging:
  - – Skeletal survey reveals lytic bone lesions in multiple myeloma.
  - – A CT pulmonary angiogram or V/Q scan is required to diagnose pulmonary embolism, whereas a leg venous Doppler may reveal deep vein thrombosis.
  - – A CT scan of the sinuses may reveal nasopharyngeal carcinoma or lesions that suggest Wegener's granulomatosis.
  - – Echocardiogram (transthoracic or transoesophageal) may reveal the characteristic vegetations of infective endocarditis.
  - – PET scan can reveal occult malignancy, infection or inflammation.
  - – An indium-labelled white cell scan may reveal occult infection such as osteomyelitis or abscess. Further nuclear medicine techniques include the gallium-67 scan (infection or malignancy) and technetium-99m scan (osteomyelitis or soft tissue abscess).
  - – Colonoscopy or flexible sigmoidoscopy may reveal inflammatory bowel disease, neutropenic or pseudomembranous colitis, diverticulitis or malignancy, whereas OGD may be diagnostic of upper gastrointestinal malignancy.

REFERENCES

1   Mackowiak PA, Durack DT. Fever of unknown origin. In: Mandell GL, Bennett JE, Dolin R (eds) *Principles and Practice of Infectious Diseases*. 6th ed. Philadelphia, PA: Elsevier; 2005. pp. 718–29.
2   Arnow PM, Flaherty JP. Fever of unknown origin. *Lancet*. 1997; **350**: 575–80.
3   Byrd WE, Hunt RE, Burgess R. Retroperitoneal fibrosis as a cause of fever of undetermined origin. *West J Med*. 1981; **134**: 357–61.
4   Papadaki HA, Kouroumalis EA, Stefanaki K *et al*. Retractile mesenteritis presenting as fever of unknown origin and autoimmune haemolytic anaemia. *Digestion*. 2000; **61**: 145–8.
5   Tsushima K, Kubo K, Kawa S *et al*. IgG4-associated multifocal systemic fibrosis presenting with fever of unknown origin. *Q J Med*. 2007; **100**: 141–2.
6   Cheng CC, Lin CY, Han CL. Intramural haematoma of the aorta presenting as fever of unknown origin. *Acta Cardiol*. 2007; **62**: 409–11.
7   Graber CJ, Lauring AS, Chin-Hong PV. A stitch in time. *NEJM*. 2007; **357**: 1029–34.

CHAPTER 31

Anaemia

PATHOPHYSIOLOGY AND AETIOLOGY

Anaemia may be defined as a blood haemoglobin concentration of less than 13.5 g/dl in men and less than 11.5 g/dl in women. It may be caused by either reduced production or increased loss of red blood cells.

Anaemia that is caused by reduced production of red blood cells may be divided into normocytic, microcytic and macrocytic types, corresponding to a mean corpuscular volume (MCV) that is low, normal and high, respectively. The normocytic group includes chronic kidney disease and the broad category of 'anaemia of chronic disease'. This is caused by chronic infection, inflammation or neoplasia. Critical illness (e.g. severe sepsis) may also cause normocytic anaemia fairly acutely. In addition, bone-marrow failure, a variety of endocrine conditions and a number of rare hereditary disorders can cause normocytic anaemia. Microcytic anaemias are usually due to iron deficiency or one of the sideroblastic anaemias. Sideroblastic anaemia refers to a group of disorders in which haem formation is defective, resulting in the formation of iron deposits in a ring around the nucleus of developing red blood cells. These so-called ringed sideroblasts may be seen in bone-marrow aspirates. Macrocytic anaemia is most often caused by vitamin deficiency, hypothyroidism or alcohol excess. Bone-marrow failure or sideroblastic anaemia may be associated with mild macrocytosis.

Increased loss of red blood cells occurs due to haemorrhage or haemolysis. Acute haemorrhage is usually associated with a normal MCV, unless there is a chronic component giving rise to concomitant iron-deficiency anaemia. Occasionally, the reticulocytosis that occurs in response to acute haemorrhage may produce a mild macrocytosis. Haemolysis is often associated with reticulocytosis and thus raised MCV. However, the underlying cause of haemolysis may itself be associated with microcytosis (e.g. thalassaemia). Thus the MCV in haemolytic anaemia varies according to the underlying cause.

The causes of anaemia are listed in Table 31.1, with common causes highlighted in bold type.

EMERGENCY MANAGEMENT

➤ The most clinically urgent cause of anaemia is acute haemorrhage. It should be noted that sudden severe haemorrhage may not cause anaemia immediately, but that this may develop later, once haemodilution has occurred.
➤ Common causes of acute haemorrhage include gastrointestinal haemorrhage, ruptured abdominal aortic aneurysm and ruptured ectopic pregnancy.
➤ Following assessment of airway and breathing, attention should be directed to the circulation. Large-bore intravenous access should be established bilaterally and blood drawn for cross-matching. If the patient is tachycardic or hypotensive, fluid resuscitation should commence with normal saline, colloid or O Rhesus-negative blood while blood is urgently cross-matched.
➤ Efforts should be directed towards stemming the source of haemorrhage. Anticoagulation should be reversed unless it is essential and, depending on the source of haemorrhage, a gastroenterologist, general surgeon, vascular surgeon or gynaecologist should be urgently consulted.

HISTORY

➤ Symptoms of anaemia include fatigue, shortness of breath and pallor. Chest pain, palpitation or syncope suggests that the anaemia is severely compromising oxygen delivery and thus requires more urgent treatment.
➤ Associated symptoms:
   – Haematemesis, coffee-ground vomiting, melaena or rectal bleeding suggest gastrointestinal haemorrhage.
   – Abdominal pain or distension may occur with intra-abdominal haemorrhage. Retroperitoneal haemorrhage (e.g. due to a ruptured abdominal aortic aneurysm) may cause loin or back pain.
   – Menorrhagia or haematuria suggests blood loss from the genital tract or urinary tract, respectively.
   – Abnormal bleeding or bruising suggests a bleeding diathesis.
   – Fever, skin rash or joint pain suggests chronic infection or inflammation.
   – Weight loss suggests underlying malignancy, and may also occur with chronic infection.
   – Dysphagia, diarrhoea, constipation or an abdominal mass may occur with gastrointestinal tract malignancy.
   – Cough and haemoptysis are features of lung cancer.
   – Jaundice and dark urine may occur with haemolysis.

Table 31.1 Causes of anaemia

Reduced production of red blood cells

Normocytic

Inflammation
► Inflammatory bowel disease
► Connective tissue disease
► Vasculitis
► Miscellaneous

Infection
► Tuberculosis
► Abscess
► Osteomyelitis
► Infective endocarditis
► Miscellaneous

Neoplasia
► Solid organ malignancy
► Lymphoma
► Lymphoproliferative disease

Endocrine and metabolic
► Chronic kidney disease
► Liver cirrhosis
► Hypothyroidism
► Hypopituitarism
► Adrenal insufficiency
► Hyperparathyroidism
► Glucagonoma
► Scurvy

Bone-marrow infiltration
► Leukaemia
► Multiple myeloma
► Metastatic infiltration
► Myelofibrosis
► Myelodysplasia
► Haemophagocytic
  lymphohistiocytosis
► Graft-versus-host disease
► Miliary tuberculosis
► Disseminated fungal infection

Microcytic

Iron deficiency
► Gastrointestinal haemorrhage
► Menorrhagia
► Idiopathic pulmonary
  haemosiderosis
► Inadequate diet

Sideroblastic anaemia

Macrocytic

Toxic, endocrine and metabolic
► Vitamin B_{12} deficiency
► Folate deficiency
► Alcohol excess
► Chronic liver disease
► Hypothyroidism

Myelodysplasia

Drugs
► Dihydrofolate reductase
  inhibitors
► Antimetabolites
► Phenytoin
► Sodium valproate
► Miscellaneous

Inherited
► Homocystinuria
► Methylmalonic aciduria
► Miscellaneous

Increased loss of red blood cells

Haemorrhage

Abdominal
► Gastrointestinal
► Abdominal aortic aneurysm
► Ectopic pregnancy
► Peripartum
► Trauma
► Miscellaneous

Extra-abdominal
► Fracture
► Vascular injury
► Soft tissue haematoma
► Haemothorax
► Pulmonary haemorrhage

Haemolysis

Red cell disorders
► Thalassaemias
► Sickle-cell anaemia
► Hereditary spherocytosis
► Hereditary elliptocytosis
► Paroxysmal nocturnal
  haemoglobinuria
► G6PD deficiency
► Pyruvate kinase deficiency
► Miscellaneous

Autoimmune
► Warm autoimmune haemolytic
  anaemia
► Cold agglutinin syndrome
► Paroxysmal cold
  haemoglobinuria
► Drug-induced haemolytic
  anaemia
► Acute haemolytic transfusion
  reaction
► Graft-versus-host disease

Microangiopathic
► TTP/HUS
► HELLP syndrome
► Malignant hypertension
► Disseminated intravascular
  coagulation
► Antiphospholipid syndrome[1]
► Miscellaneous

Mechanical
► Cardiopulmonary bypass
► Metallic heart valve
► Infective endocarditis
► Aortic stenosis[2]
► March haemoglobinuria

continued

Table 31.1 Causes of anaemia

Reduced production of red blood cells			Increased loss of red blood cells	
Normocytic	*Microcytic*	*Macrocytic*	*Haemorrhage*	*Haemolysis*
➤ Lipid storage disease				Infection
➤ Sarcoidosis				➤ Malaria
				➤ Babesiosis
Aplastic anaemia				➤ *Bartonella bacilliformis*
➤ Parvovirus B19				➤ *Clostridium perfringens*
➤ Epstein–Barr virus				➤ African trypanosomiasis
➤ Cytomegalovirus				
➤ HIV				Miscellaneous
➤ Irradiation				➤ Hypersplenism
➤ Cytotoxic drugs				➤ Acanthocytosis
➤ Paroxysmal nocturnal				➤ Megaloblastic anaemia
haemoglobinuria				➤ Congenital dyserythropoietic
➤ Hereditary				anaemia
➤ Miscellaneous				➤ Hypophosphataemia
				➤ Oxidant drugs and toxins
Miscellaneous				➤ Envenomation
➤ Anaemia of critical illness				
➤ Pure red cell aplasia				
➤ Epidermolysis bullosa				
➤ Hereditary				

➤ Drug history. Note in particular any use of antiplatelet agents, NSAIDs or anticoagulants.

EXAMINATION
➤ Check for signs of hypovolaemia, which would suggest acute haemorrhage. These include tachycardia, tachypnoea, hypotension, a postural drop in blood pressure, oliguria, confusion, cool peripheries, prolonged capillary refill time, weak thready pulse, dry mucous membranes, low JVP and reduced skin turgor.
➤ Severe anaemia may cause cardiac failure, manifested by bi-basal inspiratory crackles, raised JVP, S3 gallop rhythm and peripheral oedema.
➤ General examination:
  – Pallor may be noted with severe anaemia.
  – Fever suggests infection or inflammation.
  – Cachexia may occur with malignancy or chronic infection.
  – Lymphadenopathy suggests lymphoma or metastatic malignancy.
  – Jaundice suggests haemolysis or liver disease.
  – Palmar erythema, hepatic flap, spider naevi and gynaecomastia are signs of chronic liver disease.
  – Clubbing occurs with lung cancer, infective endocarditis, chronic liver disease and inflammatory bowel disease.
  – Splinter haemorrhages, Janaway lesions, Osler nodes and Roth spots are signs of infective endo-carditis.
  – Skin rash may occur with vasculitis or connective tissue disease.
  – Glossitis is a feature of vitamin B_{12} or folate deficiency.
➤ Abdominal examination:
  – Splenomegaly occurs with chronic infection, extravascular haemolysis, leukaemia and storage disorders.
  – Check carefully for an abdominal aortic aneurysm.
  – Palpable abdominal masses suggest solid organ malignancy.
  – Rectal examination may reveal rectal bleeding or melaena. Colorectal cancer may be palpable.
➤ Since anaemia may be associated with disease of any body system, the cardiovascular, respiratory, musculoskeletal and neurological systems must be examined carefully. Possible diagnostic clues include cardiac murmurs (infective endocarditis), joint swelling (connective tissue disease) or ataxic gait (vitamin B_{12} deficiency).

INVESTIGATIONS
The following core investigations are commonly required:
➤ Blood tests:
  – FBC and clotting screen.
  – U&Es and LFTs may indicate renal failure or hepatic dysfunction, respectively.
  – CRP and ESR are raised with chronic infection or inflammation.
  – Vitamin B_{12} and folate levels should be measured to check for deficiency.
    Ferritin, transferrin saturation and serum iron levels should be measured to check body iron stores.
➤ Urine dip may reveal microscopic haematuria, which suggests vasculitis or infective endocarditis. Gross haematuria suggests that the anaemia may be secondary to renal tract haemorrhage.
➤ CXR may reveal lung cancer or tuberculosis.
➤ OGD and/or colonoscopy are performed to investigate possible gastrointestinal haemorrhage or malignancy.

The following further investigations may be required:
➤ Blood film:
  – Sickle cells, spherocytes and elliptocytes may be seen, suggesting sickle-cell anaemia, hereditary sphe-rocytosis and hereditary elliptocytosis, respectively.
  – Pancytopaenia suggests bone-marrow failure.
  – Ring sideroblasts are seen with sideroblastic anaemia.
  – Schistocytes occur with intravascular haemolysis.
  – Reticulocytosis occurs with haemolysis or acute haemorrhage.
  – Thick and thin films should be performed if clinically indicated to search for evidence of malaria, babesiosis or *Bartonella bacilliformis* infection.
➤ Haemolysis screen:
  – LDH activity is raised with haemolysis.
  – Haptoglobin levels are low with intravascular haemolysis.
  – Direct Coomb's test is positive in immune haemolytic anaemias.
  – Haemoglobinopathy screen.
  – Ham's test is positive with paroxysmal nocturnal haemoglobinuria.

➤ Biochemistry and immunology:
  – TFTs.
  – Serum electrophoresis, serum free light chains and urinary Bence Jones protein are used to diagnose multiple myeloma.
  – An autoantibody screen (ANA, ENA, RhF and ANCA) should be requested if connective tissue disease or vasculitis is suspected clinically.
  – Intrinsic factor or parietal cell antibodies are diagnostic of pernicious anaemia.
➤ Abdominal USS or CT scan may reveal a leaking abdominal aortic aneurysm or other intra-abdominal haemorrhage. Intra-abdominal malignancy or abscess may also be seen.
➤ Bone-marrow biopsy is required to diagnose the cause of bone-marrow failure (e.g. acute leukaemia).

REFERENCES

1   Espinosa G, Bucciarelli S, Cervera R *et al.* Thrombotic microangiopathic haemolytic anaemia and antiphospholipid antibodies. *Ann Rheum Dis.* 2004; **63**: 730–6.
2   Kawase I, Matsuo T, Sasayama K *et al.* Haemolytic anaemia with aortic stenosis resolved by urgent aortic valve replacement. *Ann Thorac Surg.* 2008; **86**: 645–6.

CHAPTER 32

Skin rash

PATHOPHYSIOLOGY AND AETIOLOGY
Skin rashes may be caused by the following broad categories of mechanisms:
1 local or systemic infection
2 inflammation
3 neoplasia
4 miscellaneous causes.

Infectious and non-infectious causes of acute skin rash are listed in Tables 32.1 and 32.2, with common causes highlighted in bold type.

EMERGENCY MANAGEMENT
Although dermatology is predominantly an outpatient specialty, a small number of skin conditions may cause life-threatening systemic upset due to widespread failure of the skin to perform its essential functions, including thermoregulation and protection from infection. Fluid and electrolyte losses from the damaged skin surface may be considerable. These serious skin conditions include the following:
➤ erythroderma
➤ generalised pustular psoriasis
➤ Stevens–Johnson syndrome
➤ toxic epidermal necrolysis
➤ pemphigus
➤ eczema herpeticum.

Generic management includes regular monitoring of fluid balance and core temperature, the application of topical emollients, analgesia and the use of pressure-relieving or foam mattresses. Drugs that may have precipitated the episode should be withdrawn. Early consultation with a dermatologist is essential in order to determine the most appropriate specific treatment. For instance, eczema herpeticum is treated with IV aciclovir, whereas pemphigus requires high-dose corticosteroids.

The following life-threatening conditions may be associated with a characteristic skin rash, although the rash itself is merely a marker of the underlying disease, and not a direct cause of systemic upset:
➤ **meningococcal sepsis**: purpuric or petechial rash, classically non-blanching but may blanch in the early stages
➤ **toxic shock syndrome**: diffuse erythematous rash with subsequent desquamation
➤ **necrotising fasciitis**: deep red or purple discolouration, possibly with blistering, overlying the affected area
➤ **anaphylaxis or angioedema**: urticarial rash.

HISTORY
➤ Time of appearance of rash.
➤ Previous similar rashes.
➤ Precipitating factors:
 – sun exposure
 – recently started medications
 – new creams, lotions or washing powders
 – foods.
➤ Symptoms associated with rash:
 – pain
 – pruritus.
➤ Past medical history.
➤ Drug history:
 – Note the time at which each new medication was started.
 – Herbal, complementary and over-the-counter medications should be included.
➤ Family history.

Table 32.1 Infectious causes of acute skin rash

Viral	*Bacterial*	*Fungal*	*Miscellaneous*
Generalised rash	Local rash	Superficial skin infection	Arthropod infestation
➤ Measles	➤ Cellulitis	➤ Tinea	➤ Scabies
➤ Rubella	➤ Necrotising fasciitis	➤ Candidiasis	➤ Pediculosis
➤ Parvovirus B19	➤ Gas gangrene	➤ Pityriasis versicolor	➤ Tungosis
➤ Enteroviruses	➤ Impetigo	➤ Pityrosporum folliculitis	➤ Myiasis
➤ Chickenpox	➤ Ecthyma	➤ Scytalidium	
➤ Infectious	➤ Ecthyma gangrenosum	➤ Tinea nigra	Protozoan infection
mononucleosis	➤ Erysipelas	➤ Black piedra	➤ Cutaneous amoebiasis
➤ Cytomegalovirus	➤ Erysipeloid	➤ White piedra	➤ Cutaneous leishmaniasis
➤ HIV seroconversion	➤ Erythrasma		➤ *Balamuthia mandrillaris*
➤ HTLV-1	➤ Folliculitis	Subcutaneous infection	➤ Toxoplasmosis
➤ Dengue fever	➤ Pyoderma vegetans	➤ Mycetoma	➤ African trypanosomiasis
➤ Viral haemorrhagic fever	➤ Blistering distal dactylitis	➤ Chromoblastomycosis	➤ Chagas' disease
➤ Miscellaneous	➤ Cutaneous diphtheria	➤ Sporotrichosis	
	➤ Actinomycosis		Helminth infection
Localised rash	➤ Tuberculosis	Disseminated infection	➤ Uncinarial dermatitis
➤ Herpes simplex		➤ Aspergillosis	➤ Cercarial dermatitis
➤ Eczema herpeticum	Discrete lesions	➤ Candidiasis	➤ Katayama fever
➤ Shingles	➤ Furuncle	➤ Histoplasmosis	➤ Cutaneous larva migrans
	➤ Carbuncle	➤ Blastomycosis	➤ Visceral larva migrans
Discrete lesions	➤ Cutaneous anthrax	➤ Coccidioidomycosis	➤ Onchocerciasis
➤ Molluscum	➤ Ulceroglandular	➤ Paracoccidioidomycosis	➤ Mansonellosis
contagiosum	tularaemia	➤ Mucormycosis	➤ Dirofilariasis
➤ Warts	➤ Scrub typhus	➤ Cryptococcosis	➤ Gnathostomiasis
➤ Orf	➤ Nocardiosis	➤ Penicilliosis	➤ Trichinosis
➤ Milker's nodules	➤ Environmental		➤ Paragonimiasis
➤ Miscellaneous	mycobacteria		
	➤ Yaws		Prothecosis
	➤ Bejel		
	➤ Pinta		
	Systemic infection		
	➤ Meningococcaemia		
	➤ Gonococcaemia		
	➤ Streptococcal sepsis		
	➤ Staphylococcal sepsis		
	➤ Vibrio vulnificans sepsis		
	➤ Lyme disease		
	➤ Secondary syphilis		
	➤ Typhoid fever		
	➤ Brucellosis		
	➤ Melioidosis		
	➤ Tularaemia		
	➤ Rat bite fever		
	➤ Relapsing fever		
	➤ Leptospirosis		
	➤ Yersiniosis		
	➤ Rickettsiosis		
	➤ Bacillary angiomatosis		
	➤ Trench fever		
	➤ Cat scratch disease		
	➤ Leprosy		
	Exotoxin-mediated rash		
	➤ Toxic shock syndrome		
	➤ Staphylococcal scalded		
	skin syndrome		
	➤ Scarlet fever		

Table 32.2 Non-infectious causes of acute skin rash

Inflammation

Drug reaction

Immediate hypersensitivity
➤ Anaphylaxis
➤ Angioedema
➤ Urticaria

Blistering disorders
➤ Pemphigus
➤ Pemphigoid
➤ Erythema multiforme
➤ Stevens–Johnson
   syndrome
➤ Toxic epidermal
   necrolysis

Panniculitis
➤ Erythema nodosum
➤ α1-antitrypsin deficiency
➤ Pancreatic fat necrosis
➤ Weber–Christian disease
➤ Miscellaneous

Dermatitis
➤ Irritant contact
➤ Allergic contact

Papulosquamous disorders
➤ Erythroderma
➤ Generalised pustular
   psoriasis
➤ Acute generalised
   exanthematous
   pustulosis
➤ Pityriasis lichenoides
➤ Pityriasis rosea
➤ Transient acantholytic
   dermatosis
➤ Papuloerythroderma
➤ Papular pruritic eruption
➤ Polymorphic light
   eruption

Dermatoses of pregnancy
➤ Atopic eruption of
   pregnancy
➤ Polymorphic eruption
   of pregnancy
➤ Pemphigoid gestationis

Collagen vascular disease
➤ Systemic lupus
   erythematosus
➤ Rheumatoid arthritis
➤ Mixed connective
   tissue disease
➤ Adult Still's disease
➤ Dermatomyositis
➤ Reactive arthritis
➤ SAPHO syndrome

Vasculitis
➤ Henoch–Schönlein
   purpura
➤ Cutaneous
   leukocytoclastic vasculitis
➤ Wegener's
   granulomatosis
➤ Churg–Strauss syndrome
➤ Microscopic polyangiitis
➤ Polyarteritis nodosa
➤ Drug-induced vasculitis
➤ Cryoglobulinaemia
➤ Behçet's disease
➤ Kawasaki disease

Miscellaneous
➤ Sarcoidosis
➤ Rheumatic fever
➤ Pyoderma gangrenosum
➤ Acute interstitial nephritis
➤ Familial periodic fevers
➤ Serum sickness
➤ Kikuchi disease
➤ Fibroblastic rheumatism
➤ Sweet's syndrome
➤ Eosinophilic cellulitis
➤ Malakoplakia
➤ Graft versus host
   disease
➤ Engraftment syndrome
➤ Eosinophilic folliculitis
➤ Eosinophilia-myalgia
   syndrome

Neoplasia

Cutaneous metastases

Lymphoproliferative
disorders
➤ Cutaneous lymphoma
➤ Intravascular lymphoma
➤ Angioimmunoblastic
   lymphadenopathy with
   dysproteinaemia
➤ Lymphomatoid
   granulomatosis
➤ POEMS syndrome

Histiocytoses
➤ Langerhans cell
   histiocytosis
➤ Erdheim–Chester
   disease
➤ Haemophagocytic
   lymphohistiocytosis
➤ Multicentric
   reticulohistiocytosis
➤ Malignant histiocytosis

Miscellaneous
➤ Hypereosinophilia
   syndrome
➤ Mastocytosis
➤ Leukaemia cutis

Miscellaneous

Toxins
➤ Heavy metal toxicity
➤ Scombrotoxic fish
   poisoning

Nutrient deficiency
➤ Scurvy
➤ Pellagra
➤ Zinc deficiency

Environmental injury
➤ Temperature extremes
➤ Chemical
➤ Irradiation
➤ Bites and stings
➤ Envenomation

Vascular
➤ Endocarditis
➤ Septic emboli
➤ Atrial myxoma
➤ Cholesterol embolism
➤ Decompression sickness
➤ Sneddon's syndrome
➤ Antiphospholipid
   syndrome
➤ Livedoid vasculopathy
➤ Livedo reticularis
➤ Degos' disease
➤ Calciphylaxis
➤ Warfarin-induced skin
   necrosis
➤ Thrombocytopaenia
➤ Platelet dysfunction

Paraneoplastic
➤ Erythema gyratum
   repens
➤ Acanthosis nigricans
➤ Acrokeratosis
   neoplastica
➤ Necrolytic migratory
   erythema

Blistering disorders
➤ Cutaneous porphyrias
➤ Pseudoporphyria
➤ Bullosis diabeticorum

Miscellaneous
➤ Amyloidosis
➤ Eruptive xanthoma
➤ Erythema annulare
   centrifugum

➤ Social history:
  – foreign travel
  – occupation
  – hobbies.

EXAMINATION

The diagnosis of skin rashes largely relies on experience and pattern recognition. As the number of possible skin rashes is vast, the reader is referred to specialised dermatology textbooks for detailed descriptions and photographs of the various conditions that may be encountered. In general, the following features should be elicited during the clinical examination:

➤ Distribution of rash:
  – symmetrical or asymmetrical
  – central or peripheral
  – flexor or extensor surfaces of limbs involved
  – confined to sun-exposed areas
  – widespread or circumscribed.
➤ Appearance and texture of rash:
  – nature of the lesion(s) (e.g. macules, patches, nodules, papules, plaques, weals, vesicles, bullae or pustules)
  – colour, size and shape of lesions
  – scales or crusts suggest epidermal involvement (e.g. due to psoriasis or impetigo), whereas normal skin texture suggests a dermal lesion (e.g. erythema nodosum).
➤ Inspect the nails:
  – Splinter haemorrhages occur with vasculitis and infective endocarditis.
  – Clubbing is a further feature of infective endocarditis.
  – Pitting is seen with psoriasis.

INVESTIGATIONS

The following investigations may be required:
➤ Blood tests:
  – FBC and CRP should be performed to check for evidence of systemic inflammation.
  – An autoimmune screen is indicated in cases of suspected vasculitis or connective tissue disease. This includes ANA, anti-dsDNA (SLE), RhF (rheumatoid arthritis), ANCA (Churg–Strauss syndrome, Wegener's granulomatosis), anti-Jo-1 (dermatomyositis), anti-RNP (mixed connective tissue disease), anti-cardiolipin antibodies and lupus anticoagulant (anti-phospholipid syndrome), and cryoglobulins.
  – Mast cell tryptase activity is raised following anaphylaxis.
  – Levels of C2 and C4 complement components, and C1 esterase inhibitor, are low in hereditary angioedema.
➤ Microbiology:
  – Blood culture should be performed if sepsis is suspected clinically.
  – Microscopy of skin scrapings may reveal fungal hyphae or parasites.
  – Viral serology should be performed for EBV, HSV, VZV, HIV, measles and rubella if clinically indicated.
  – Bacterial serology may be performed for Lyme disease or brucellosis. The TPHA or VDRL test should be performed for treponemal infection (syphilis, yaws, bejel, pinta). Anti-streptolysin O titre is raised with recent streptococcal infection.
➤ Skin biopsy may be required to make the diagnosis.

CHAPTER 33

Acid–base disturbances

INTRODUCTION

The clinical importance of acid–base assessment is twofold. First, the regulation of acid–base balance is essential for normal cellular functioning. Secondly, the analysis of acid–base disturbances can provide important diagnostic information about the underlying condition. The acid–base status of a patient should not be considered in isolation, but rather it should be viewed in the context of the overall clinical presentation. The history and examination should be tailored to the patient's presenting complaint. Acid–base status is assessed by sampling arterial or venous blood and measuring the pH, pCO_2 and bicarbonate concentration ($[HCO_3^-]$). The normal ranges of these parameters are as follows:

pH	7.35–7.45
pCO_2	4.8–6.1 kPa
$[HCO_3^-]$	22–28 mmol/l.

An acidosis is any primary process that tends to reduce the pH, whereas an alkalosis is any primary process that tends to increase the pH. Acid–base disturbances caused by changes in pCO_2 are referred to as respiratory, whereas disturbances caused by changes in the concentration of other chemical species are referred to as metabolic. Acids other than carbon dioxide are sometimes referred to as 'fixed acids', as they cannot be excreted by the respiratory system, and are instead metabolised or excreted by the kidneys.

The following chemical equilibrium exists in plasma:

$$H_2O + CO_2 \longleftrightarrow HCO_3^- + H^+$$

Any increase in the pCO_2 pushes the equilibrium to the right, thus lowering the pH, whereas a fall in the pCO_2 pulls the equilibrium to the left, thus raising the pH. Similarly, an increase in the HCO_3^- concentration pushes the equilibrium to the left, thus raising the pH, whereas a fall in the HCO_3^- concentration pulls the equilibrium to the right, thus lowering the pH.

This may be represented mathematically using the modified Henderson equation:

$$[H^+] = k \times pCO_2/[HCO_3^-]$$

where k is a constant.

STANDARD BASE EXCESS

Whereas the pCO_2 reliably indicates the extent of the respiratory component of an acid–base disorder, the metabolic component is more difficult to quantify, as the HCO_3^- concentration is affected by both respiratory and metabolic disturbances.

The standard base excess (SBE) provides the most reliable measure of the net metabolic component of a patient's acid–base status. It is a calculated value that estimates the quantity of base that would be necessary to return the pH to 7.4, assuming that the pCO_2 was 5.3 kPa (i.e. assuming that there was no respiratory acidosis or alkalosis). The normal range of SBE is –2 to +2 mEq/l. A negative SBE indicates a net metabolic acidosis or metabolic compensation for a primary respiratory alkalosis, whereas a positive SBE indicates a net metabolic alkalosis or metabolic compensation for a primary respiratory acidosis. However, the base excess may be normal in the presence of a metabolic acidosis and metabolic alkalosis that cancel each other out.

It should be noted that the SBE does not distinguish between primary metabolic acid–base disturbances and metabolic compensation for respiratory acid–base disturbances. Thus a patient with chronic type II respiratory failure with metabolic compensation will have a positive base excess. However, by convention a compensatory response to a primary acid–base disturbance is not referred to as an acidosis or alkalosis, as such compensation is a normal physiological process.

COMPENSATORY RESPONSES TO ACID–BASE DISTURBANCES

In normal circumstances, a primary respiratory acid–base disturbance will be accompanied by metabolic compensation, mediated by the kidneys, that tends to return the pH towards normal. Specifically, a respiratory acidosis will be compensated for by excretion of Cl⁻ and retention of HCO_3^- by the kidney, while a respiratory alkalosis will be compensated for by renal retention of Cl⁻ and excretion of HCO_3^-. Maximal compensation may take several days to occur, thus allowing a distinction to be made between acute and chronic respiratory acid–base disturbances.

Similarly, a primary metabolic acid–base disturbance will be accompanied by respiratory compensation that tends to return the pH towards normal. Specifically, a metabolic acidosis will cause compensatory hyperventilation, thus reducing the pCO_2, whereas a metabolic alkalosis may result in a degree of hypoventilation, thus increasing the pCO_2. Maximal compensation may take a number of hours.

There are a number of simple rules that allow the estimation of the magnitude of compensation that may be expected for any given acid–base disorder. These rules have been derived from empirical studies of patients with acid–base disturbances. Deviation from the expected level of compensation implies that a second primary acid–base disturbance is likely to be occurring – that is, that the patient has a mixed acid–base disorder. A useful rule of thumb is that if the pCO_2 and HCO_3^- concentration move in opposite directions, a mixed acid–base disorder must be present, although the converse of this does not always hold. Table 33.1 shows the changes that may be expected in each primary acid–base disorder.

Table 33.1 Expected blood gas changes in primary acid–base disorders[1,2]

Acid–base disorder	pH	pCO_2	$[HCO_3^-]$	Compensation rule
Acute respiratory acidosis	↓	↑	↑	$[HCO_3^-]$ ↑ by 1 mmol/l above 24 mmol/l for every 1 kPa rise in pCO_2 above 5.3 kPa
Chronic respiratory acidosis	↓	↑	↑	$[HCO_3^-]$ ↑ by 4 mmol/l above 24 mmol/l for every 1 kPa rise in pCO_2 above 5.3 kPa
Acute respiratory alkalosis	↑	↓	↓	$[HCO_3^-]$ ↓ by 2 mmol/l below 24 mmol/l for every 1 kPa fall in pCO_2 below 5.3 kPa
Chronic respiratory alkalosis	↑	↓	↓	$[HCO_3^-]$ ↓ by 3 mmol/l below 24 mmol/l for every 1 kPa fall in pCO_2 below 5.3 kPa
Metabolic acidosis	↓	↓	↓	$pCO_2 = [HCO_3^-]/5 + 1.1$
Metabolic alkalosis	↑	↑	↑	$pCO_2 = [HCO_3^-]/11 + 2.8$

RESPIRATORY ACID–BASE DISTURBANCES

Respiratory acidosis is caused by reduced alveolar ventilation, which leads to a raised pCO_2. This may result from either respiratory or neuromuscular disease, as shown in Table 33.2. Conversely, respiratory alkalosis is caused by increased alveolar ventilation, leading to a reduced pCO_2. This may result from primary respiratory centre dysfunction or from stimulation of the respiratory centre by hypoxia or other factors, as shown in Table 33.3.

Table 33.2 Causes of respiratory acidosis

Respiratory disease	*Neuromuscular disease*

Respiratory disease

Airway disease
➤ COPD
➤ Asthma
➤ Obstructive sleep apnoea

Upper airway obstruction
➤ Anaphylaxis
➤ Angioedema
➤ Mastocytosis
➤ Epiglottitis
➤ Diphtheria
➤ Inhaled foreign body
➤ Tracheal stenosis
➤ Tumour
➤ Vocal cord dysfunction or paralysis
➤ Extrinsic compression

Chest wall or pleural disease
➤ Scoliosis/kyphoscoliosis
➤ Ankylosing spondylitis
➤ Chest trauma
➤ Thoracic surgery
➤ Diffuse pleural thickening
➤ Malignant mesothelioma

Reduced lung compliance
➤ Pulmonary oedema
➤ ARDS

Neuromuscular disease

Respiratory centre depression
➤ Obesity hypoventilation
➤ Central sleep apnoea
➤ Ethanol
➤ Benzodiazepines
➤ Opiates
➤ Barbiturates
➤ Brainstem damage
➤ Hypothyroidism

High cervical spinal cord injury

Peripheral neuropathy
➤ Guillain–Barré syndrome
➤ CIDP
➤ Motor neuron disease
➤ Multifocal motor neuropathy
➤ Charcot–Marie–Tooth disease
➤ Critical illness polyneuropathy
➤ Bilateral diaphragm paralysis
➤ Poliomyelitis
➤ Acute porphyria
➤ Miscellaneous

Neuromuscular junction blockade
➤ Myasthenia gravis
➤ LEMS
➤ Botulism
➤ Marine neurotoxins
➤ Tick paralysis
➤ Envenomation
➤ Organophosphates

Increased muscle tone
➤ Tetanus
➤ Strychnine poisoning
➤ Neuroleptic malignant syndrome
➤ Status dystonicus

Myopathy
➤ Muscular dystrophy
➤ Myotonic dystrophy
➤ Polymyositis
➤ Dermatomyositis
➤ Acid maltase deficiency
➤ Hypophosphataemia
➤ Miscellaneous

METABOLIC ACIDOSIS

The requirement for electrical neutrality of the plasma dictates that the electrical charge of the cations in solution (measured in mEq/l) must equal that of the anions, as shown in the following equation:

$$[Na^+] + [K^+] + [Ca^{2+}] + [Mg^{2+}] = [Cl^-] + [HCO_3^-] + [PO_4^{3-}] + [Alb^-] + [XA^-]$$

where [Alb⁻] represents negative charges on albumin, and [XA⁻] represents other anions that may be present in abnormal quantities, such as lactate and ketone bodies.

All other things being equal, an increase in Cl⁻ concentration is necessarily associated with a reduction in HCO_3^- concentration in order to maintain electrical neutrality. As shown by the modified Henderson equation, this causes a metabolic acidosis, known as hyperchloraemic acidosis. Similarly, an abnormal increase in anions such as lactate (lactic acidosis), ketone bodies (ketoacidosis) or metabolites of ingested poisons, such as volatile alcohols, results in metabolic acidosis. Critically ill patients, such as those with shock or sepsis, have sometimes been observed to have a metabolic acidosis that could not be explained by raised

Table 33.3 Causes of respiratory alkalosis

Respiratory centre stimulation	*Respiratory centre damage*
Reduced blood oxygen carriage	Head injury
➤ Hypoxia	
➤ Anaemia	Brainstem infarction
➤ Carbon monoxide poisoning	
	Brainstem haemorrhage
Pulmonary conditions	
➤ Asthma	Meningitis
➤ Pulmonary embolism	
	Encephalitis
Psychogenic	
➤ Hyperventilation syndrome	Tumour
➤ Panic attack	
➤ Anxiety	
➤ Pain	
Drugs and toxins	
➤ Salicylate poisoning	
➤ Nicotine	
➤ Progesterone	
➤ Methylxanthines	
➤ Catecholamines	
Miscellaneous	
➤ Hyperthyroidism	
➤ Hepatic failure	
➤ Sepsis	
➤ Fever	
➤ Pregnancy	

levels of lactate or any other easily measured anion. Increased levels of Krebs cycle intermediates may account for the acidosis in some cases.[3] Hyperalbuminaemia is uncommon, but when it occurs a mild metabolic acidosis results, since albumin is a weak acid.

Dilutional acidosis is a further independent mechanism of metabolic acidosis. An excess of free water will dilute all components of the plasma equally, thus moving the pH closer to 7, which is the pH of pure water. As the normal pH of plasma is approximately 7.4, the addition of free water will thus cause a so-called dilutional acidosis.

Metabolic acidosis due to chloride excess may be distinguished from that due to an excess of other anions by calculating the anion gap (AG). This is defined as the difference between the total concentration (in mEq/l) of the commonly measured cations and that of the commonly measured anions in the plasma:

$$AG = [Na^+] + [K^+] - [HCO_3^-] - [Cl^-].$$

Thus the anion gap is a measure of the magnitude of the concentration of unmeasured anions in the plasma over and above that of unmeasured cations. The concentration of unmeasured anions (Alb^-, PO_4^{3-} and XA^-) generally exceeds that of unmeasured cations (Mg^{2+} and Ca^{2+}) by approximately 15–20 mEq/l, and therefore this is the normal range of the anion gap. Metabolic acidosis due to chloride excess will not alter the anion gap, as chloride is one of the measured anions. However, metabolic acidosis due to an excess of other anions, such as lactate or ketone bodies, will result in a raised anion gap. It should be noted that significant hypoalbuminaemia may lower the anion gap and so mask the diagnosis of a metabolic acidosis due to unmeasured anions. Thus, in cases of hypoalbuminaemia, the corrected anion gap should be calculated using the following formula:[4]

$$AG_{corr} = AG + (40 - [Alb (g/l)])/4.$$

The causes of metabolic acidosis may be conveniently classified according to whether the anion gap is normal or raised, as shown in Table 33.4.

The osmolal gap is the difference between the measured and the calculated osmolality of serum, where:

calculated osmolality $= 2 \times [Na^+] + [glucose] + [urea]$.

Table 33.4 Causes of metabolic acidosis[5]

Normal anion gap	Raised anion gap
Chloride administration	Ketoacidosis
	➤ Diabetic
	➤ Alcoholic
Loss of low-chloride fluid	➤ Starvation
➤ Diarrhoea	
➤ Pancreatic fistula or drain	
➤ Biliary fistula or drain	Lactic acidosis
➤ Ureteroenterostomy	➤ Shock
	➤ Sepsis
Renal chloride retention (drug induced)	➤ Hypoxia
➤ ACE inhibitors	➤ Mesenteric or limb ischaemia
➤ Angiotensin-receptor antagonists	➤ Fulminant hepatic failure
➤ Potassium-sparing diuretics	➤ Pancreatitis
➤ Acetazolamide	➤ Seizure
➤ NSAIDs	➤ Alcohol intoxication
➤ Miscellaneous	➤ Carbon monoxide poisoning
	➤ Paracetamol poisoning
Renal chloride retention (non-drug induced)	➤ Biguanides
➤ Proximal renal tubular acidosis	➤ Miscellaneous
➤ Distal renal tubular acidosis	
➤ Hyporeninaemic hypoaldosteronism	Renal failure
➤ Mineralocorticoid synthetic defects	
➤ Pseudohypoaldosteronism	Poisoning
	➤ Salicylates
Dilutional acidosis	➤ Ethylene glycol
	➤ Ethanol
	➤ Methanol
	➤ Paraldehyde
	➤ Solvent abuse
	Miscellaneous
	➤ Critical illness[3]
	➤ Hyperphosphataemia
	➤ Hyperalbuminaemia
	➤ Rhabdomyolysis
	➤ Tumour lysis syndrome
	➤ Total parenteral nutrition
	➤ Pyroglutamic acidaemia
	➤ Urea cycle disorders
	➤ Amino acid metabolism disorders
	➤ Fatty acid oxidation disorders

The normal range for the osmolal gap is 10–15 mOsm/kg. A value higher than this implies the presence of a significant quantity of unmeasured osmotically active solutes. Therefore the osmolal gap is a useful diagnostic tool for the investigation of unexplained high anion gap metabolic acidosis. The commonest cause of an elevated osmolal gap in clinical practice is poisoning by volatile alcohols.

Investigations that may be required to diagnose a metabolic acidosis include the following:
➤ Urine dip. The presence of glucose and ketones suggests diabetic ketoacidosis.
➤ Blood tests:
  – U&Es and PO_4^{3-} may reveal renal failure and/or hyperphosphataemia.
  – LFT derangement, raised INR and low albumin levels are features of hepatic failure.
  – Glucose levels are elevated in diabetic ketoacidosis.
  – Lactate.
  – Urate levels are raised in tumour lysis syndrome.
  – Creatine kinase activity is raised with rhabdomyolysis.
  – Amylase activity should be checked if pancreatitis is a clinical possibility.
  – Serum ammonia levels are raised with hepatic failure, urea cycle disorders and disorders of amino acid metabolism.
➤ Toxicology screen (salicylates, paracetamol, ethanol, methanol and ethylene glycol).

Table 33.5 Causes of metabolic alkalosis[6-9]

Renal chloride loss	Extra-renal chloride loss	Alkali load	Miscellaneous
Mineralocorticoid excess	Gastrointestinal	Milk-alkali syndrome	Contraction alkalosis
	➤ Vomiting		Hypoalbuminaemia
Miscellaneous	➤ **Nasogastric suction**	Bicarbonate infusion	
Drugs	➤ Laxative abuse	Blood transfusion	
➤ **Loop diuretics**	➤ Congenital chloridorrhoea		
➤ **Thiazide diuretics**	➤ Miscellaneous	Haemodialysis	
➤ Penicillin		Refeeding syndrome	
Exogenous mineralocorticoid	Cutaneous		
➤ **Corticosteroids**	➤ Cystic fibrosis	Post-lactic acidosis or ketoacidosis	
➤ **Fludrocortisone**	➤ Excessive sweating		
Renin-mediated mineralocorticoid excess			
Post-hypercapnia			
➤ **Renovascular disease**			
➤ Renal artery stenosis			
Hypokalaemia			
➤ Renin-secreting tumour			
➤ Malignant hypertension			
Hypercalcaemia			
ACTH-mediated mineralocorticoid excess	Inherited tubular disorders		
➤ ACTH-producing pituitary adenoma	➤ Bartter's syndrome		
	➤ Liddle's syndrome		
➤ Glucocorticoid resistance[7]	➤ Gitelman's syndrome		
➤ Glucocorticoid-remediable aldosteronism			
Primary mineralocorticoid excess			
➤ Conn's syndrome			
➤ Cushing's disease			
➤ Deoxycorticosterone-secreting tumour			
➤ 11-β-hydroxylase deficiency			
➤ 17-α-hydroxylase deficiency			
11-β-hydroxysteroid dehydrogenase type 2 inactivity			
➤ Syndrome of apparent mineralocorticoid excess			
➤ Carbenoxolone			
➤ Chewing tobacco			
➤ Liquorice excess			
Activating mineralocorticoid receptor mutation[8]			

METABOLIC ALKALOSIS

Due to the requirement for electrical neutrality of plasma, a reduction in Cl^- concentration is necessarily associated with a rise in HCO_3^- concentration and thus a metabolic alkalosis. Chloride loss may occur via the kidneys, gastrointestinal tract or skin. Renal chloride loss most commonly occurs as a result of diuretic therapy, but additional causes include mineralocorticoid excess, severe hypokalaemia and inherited tubular disorders.

Metabolic compensation for chronic respiratory acidosis is a normal phenomenon. However, if the respiratory disorder is corrected rapidly, a transient metabolic alkalosis may occur until the HCO_3^- concentration returns to the normal level. This is known as post-hypercapnic alkalosis.[6]

The administration or endogenous production of alkali will result in metabolic alkalosis, as will hypoalbuminaemia, since albumin is a weak acid. Because plasma is normally slightly alkaline by comparison with pure water, a deficit of free water results in a metabolic alkalosis, as the plasma is literally more concentrated. This is known as contraction alkalosis.

The causes of metabolic alkalosis are summarised in Table 33.5.

The examination of a patient with metabolic alkalosis should focus on the blood pressure and volume status. Hypertension is associated with mineralocorticoid excess and Liddle's syndrome. The other causes of renal chloride loss lead to hypovolaemia, as does chloride loss from the gastrointestinal tract or skin. Specific clinical features that are seen with Cushing's syndrome include centripetal obesity, buffalo hump, moon face, abdominal striae, plethora and proximal muscle wasting. Chronic vomiting due to bulimia or anorexia nervosa may lead to dental caries and parotid enlargement. Additional signs of anorexia nervosa include low body mass index and lanugo hair. Abdominal examination may reveal a flank mass representing a renin-secreting renal-cell carcinoma or an abdominal bruit due to renal artery stenosis.

The following investigations may be required to diagnose a metabolic alkalosis:

➤ U&Es and calcium levels may reveal hypokalaemia or hypercalcaemia.
➤ Urinary electrolytes may be of diagnostic value in distinguishing between renal and extra-renal chloride loss. A urinary Cl^- concentration of < 10 mEq/l suggests extra-renal chloride loss.[9]
➤ Plasma renin and aldosterone levels may be helpful in distinguishing between the various causes of mineralocorticoid excess. For example, Conn's syndrome causes low renin and high aldosterone levels, whereas renovascular disease causes elevated levels of both renin and aldosterone.
➤ The 24-hour urinary free cortisol or dexamethasone suppression test is used to diagnose Cushing's syndrome.
➤ Inherited tubular disorders each have a characteristic pattern of urinary electrolyte abnormalities. Urinary Na+, K+, Mg^{2+} and Ca^{2+} levels may be checked if clinically indicated. Definitive diagnosis requires genetic analysis.
➤ Urinary diuretic and/or laxative screen is necessary if occult ingestion is suspected.
➤ USS, CT or MR angiography may reveal renal artery stenosis or a hormone-secreting renal or adrenal tumour.

REFERENCES

1 Baillie JK. Simple, easily memorised 'rules of thumb' for the rapid assessment of physiological compensation for respiratory acid–base disorders. *Thorax.* 2008; **63**: 289–90.
2 Kellum JA. Clinical review: reunification of acid–base physiology. *Crit Care.* 2005; **9**: 500–7.
3 Forni LG, McKinnon W, Hilton PJ. Unmeasured anions in metabolic acidosis: unravelling the mystery. *Crit Care.* 2006; **10**: 220.
4 Figge J, Jabor A, Kazda A *et al.* Anion gap and hypoalbuminemia. *Crit Care Med.* 1998; **26**: 1807–10.
5 Morris CG, Low J. Metabolic acidosis in the critically ill. Part 2. Causes and treatment. *Anaesthesia.* 2008; **63**: 396–411.
6 Palmer BF, Narins RG, Yee J. Clinical acid–base disorders. In: Davison AM, Cameron SJ, Grünfeld J *et al.* (eds) *Oxford Textbook of Clinical Nephrology.* 3rd ed. Oxford: Oxford University Press; 2005. pp. 321–43.
7 Charmandari E, Kino T, Ichijo T *et al.* Generalized glucocorticoid resistance: clinical aspects, molecular mechanisms and implications of a rare genetic disorder. *J Clin Endocrinol Metab.* 2008; **93**: 1563–72.
8 Geller DS, Farhi A, Pinkerton N *et al.* Activating mineralocorticoid receptor mutation in hypertension exacerbated by pregnancy. *Science.* 2000; **289**: 119–23.
9 Galla JH. Metabolic alkalosis. *J Am Soc Nephrol.* 2000; **11**: 369–75.

CHAPTER 34

Hyponatraemia

PATHOPHYSIOLOGY AND AETIOLOGY

Hyponatraemia is defined as a serum sodium concentration of less than 135 mmol/l. It arises due to an imbalance between the sodium and water content of the extracellular fluid, with a relative excess of water. Severe hyponatraemia, especially of acute onset, may be life-threatening due to the resulting cerebral oedema. Hyponatraemia may arise by three main mechanisms, each of which is described below.

Hypotonic hyponatraemia

The majority of cases of hyponatraemia are caused by an excess of total body water relative to total body sodium. This excess water is distributed equally throughout all of the body compartments, thus lowering the concentration of all solutes and resulting in hyponatraemia with a low serum osmolality.

Hypotonic hyponatraemia should be considered a disorder primarily of water balance rather than of sodium balance. Most of the total body sodium is kept within the extracellular compartment by Na^+/K^+ antiporters on cell membranes. Any increase or decrease in the total body sodium is accompanied by the movement of water into or out of the extracellular compartment, respectively, due to solute drag. Thus changes in total body sodium mainly affect the extracellular volume, with less prominent effects on the extracellular Na^+ concentration and osmolality.

The independence of sodium and water balance is highlighted by the fact that they are regulated by two separate endocrine control mechanisms. Sodium balance, and thus extracellular volume, is controlled by the renin–angiotensin system (RAS), whereas water balance, and thus body fluid osmolality, is controlled by the ADH–thirst axis. Hypotonic hyponatraemia may thus occur in association with low, normal or high total body sodium, corresponding to hypovolaemia, euvolaemia or hypervolaemia, respectively.

Hypovolaemic states

Any cause of hypovolaemia may be accompanied by hyponatraemia. This occurs because the ADH–thirst axis, although primarily responsible for regulating body fluid osmolality, may also be activated by extreme hypovolaemia. In this circumstance, free water is retained in order to bolster the effective arterial blood volume (EABV). Thus such non-osmotic ADH release serves to maintain EABV at the expense of a reduction in osmolality.

Euvolaemic states

A pure excess of free water without derangement of sodium balance may occur as a result of a primary increase in water intake. This may occur acutely (e.g. in marathon runners or nightclub revellers) or more chronically (often in association with psychological morbidity and compulsive water drinking). A second large group is caused by the syndrome of inappropriate ADH secretion (SIADH), in which a variety of cerebral or pulmonary pathologies may result in an increase in ADH production. Other miscellaneous causes include hypothyroidism and inadequate diets that contain insufficient electrolytes (e.g. the 'tea and toast' diet eaten by some elderly people, or the consumption of beer almost to the exclusion of all else). Decreased electrolyte intake reduces the excretion of free water by the kidneys.[1]

Hypervolaemic states

Patients with cardiac failure activate both the RAS and the ADH–thirst axis in order to maximise preload and thus cardiac output. The end result is a combination of hypervolaemia and hyponatraemia. Some hypoalbuminaemic states, such as nephrotic syndrome and liver cirrhosis, also cause activation of both the RAS and ADH–thirst axis in an attempt to boost the EABV. This is because hypoalbuminaemia reduces the oncotic pressure that normally prevents fluid from leaking out of the circulation into the interstitium. As a result, fluid exits the circulation, causing oedema and at the same time leaving the intravascular compartment depleted. Finally, acute or chronic renal failure may be associated with a failure to excrete excess sodium and excess free water, resulting in hypervolaemia and hyponatraemia.

Non-hypotonic hyponatraemia

The presence of an abnormal osmotically active solute, accompanied by water, within the serum will result in dilution of other solutes, such as sodium, thus resulting in hyponatraemia without a low serum osmolality. Non-hypotonic hyponatraemia is most commonly caused by hyperglycaemia. Other causes include mannitol infusion or the systemic absorption of iso-osmotic or hyper-osmotic solutions used for irrigation of the bladder, colon, uterus or peritoneal cavity. Finally, critically ill patients may develop generalised cellular dysfunction, known as the sick cell syndrome, in which solutes leak out of cells into the extracellular space, thus exerting an osmotic effect and resulting in non-hypotonic hyponatraemia.

Pseudohyponatraemia
Pseudohyponatraemia is a measurement error caused by an increase in the levels of plasma proteins or lipids, resulting in a proportional reduction in the aqueous component of plasma, in which sodium is dissolved. This results in a falsely low measured sodium concentration, despite the fact that the concentration in the aqueous phase of plasma is normal.

The causes of hyponatraemia are listed in Table 34.1, with common causes highlighted in bold type.

EMERGENCY MANAGEMENT
Excessively rapid correction of hyponatraemia may result in central pontine myelinolysis (CPN), a potentially fatal condition caused by CNS demyelination that occurs as a result of rapid changes in extracellular osmolality. The risk of CPN is higher in patients with chronic hyponatraemia, whereas patients with acute hyponatraemia are at greater risk of cerebral oedema due to the hyponatraemia itself. The rate of correction of hyponatraemia should take into account the likely speed of onset (most cases are chronic), and the presence or absence of neurological signs such as seizures or coma. The rate of correction should not exceed 12 mmol/l per day. Therefore aim for a maximum rate of 8 mmol/l per day initially in order to maintain a safety margin. However, if seizures or coma are present, the Na⁺ concentration should be increased by approximately 6 mmol/l over the first 3–4 hours.[2] Such an increase is usually sufficient to correct neurological features. During the treatment of severe hyponatraemia, the serum sodium concentration should be measured every 2–4 hours to ensure that the rate of correction is not too fast or too slow. Once a safe level (120 mmol/l) has been reached, the rate of correction should be more gradual. A completely normal Na⁺ concentration should not be aimed for initially.

The treatment modality that is utilised depends on the cause of hyponatraemia.
1   Hyponatraemia with hypovolaemia should be treated with intravenous normal saline in order to restore extracellular volume and thus abolish non-osmotic ADH release.
2   Hyponatraemia with euvolaemia is treated with fluid restriction initially. If this is unsuccessful, demeclocycline may be given in order to produce a state of renal insensitivity to the action of ADH.
3   Hyponatraemia with hypervolaemia is treated with salt and water restriction, and diuretics.
4   In symptomatic patients in whom more rapid correction is required, such as a patient who has acute hyponatraemia with seizures, hypertonic (3%) saline may be used under expert supervision with close monitoring. This is rarely required in day-to-day practice, and there is a risk of precipitating central pontine myelinolysis if hypertonic saline is used inappropriately. However, in selected cases it may be life-saving. The following formula may be used to calculate the expected change in serum sodium concentration produced by the infusion of 1 litre of a given concentration of saline:[3]

$$\text{change in serum } [Na^+] = \frac{\text{infusate } [Na^+] - \text{serum } [Na^+]}{\text{total body water} + 1}$$

where total body water (l) = body weight (kg) × correction factor.

Correction factors are as follows:

non-elderly man:	0.60
non-elderly woman:	0.50
elderly man:	0.50
elderly woman:	0.45

A 0.9 % solution of sodium chloride contains 154 mmol/l of sodium, whereas 3% sodium chloride contains 513 mmol/l of sodium.

5   Medications that are known to cause hyponatraemia should be stopped if possible.

HISTORY
➤ Clinical features of cerebral oedema include nausea, vomiting, drowsiness, confusion, headache and seizures.
➤ Thirst suggests hypovolaemia, whereas oedema, orthopnoea and paroxysmal nocturnal dyspnoea occur with hypervolaemia.
➤ Cough and dyspnoea suggest pulmonary disease, possibly causing SIADH.
➤ Drug history. Note any use of loop or thiazide diuretics, SSRIs or other drugs that may cause hyponatraemia.

Table 34.1 Causes of hyponatraemia

Hypotonic hyponatraemia				Non-hypotonic hyponatraemia	Pseudo-hyponatraemia
Hypovolaemic	*Euvolaemic*	*Hypervolaemic*	*Miscellaneous*		
	SIADH				
Renal sodium loss	Pulmonary	Cardiac failure	Intravenous fluid therapy	Hyperglycaemia	Hyperlipidaemia
➤ Diuretics	➤ **Bronchial carcinoma**	Renal failure	Primary polydipsia	Mannitol infusion	Plasma cell dyscrasias
➤ Salt-wasting nephropathy	➤ **Pneumonia**	Nephrotic syndrome	Hypothyroidism	Fluid irrigation	
➤ Adrenal insufficiency	➤ Lung abscess	Liver cirrhosis	Reset osmostat	➤ Bladder	
	➤ Empyema			➤ Uterine	
Extra-renal sodium loss	➤ Tuberculosis		Stress	➤ Colonic	
➤ **Diarrhoea**	➤ Miscellaneous			➤ Laparoscopic	
➤ **Vomiting**			Reduced electrolyte intake		
➤ Burns	Intracranial			Sick cell syndrome	
➤ Excessive sweating	➤ **Thromboembolic stroke**				
	➤ **Haemorrhage**				
Fluid sequestration	➤ Tumour				
➤ Bowel obstruction	➤ Cerebral abscess				
➤ Ileus	➤ Head injury				
➤ Ascites	➤ Pituitary surgery				
➤ Pancreatitis	➤ Encephalitis				
	➤ Meningitis				
	➤ Miscellaneous				
	Drugs				
	➤ **SSRIs**				
	➤ Antipsychotics				
	➤ Chlorpropamide				
	➤ Carbamazepine				
	➤ Desmopressin				
	➤ NSAIDs				
	➤ Miscellaneous				
	Miscellaneous				
	➤ Solid organ malignancy				
	➤ Acute porphyria				

➤ Enquire about illicit drug use. Ecstasy has been associated with deaths due to polydipsia and acute severe hyponatraemia.

EXAMINATION
➤ Assessment of volume status is a crucial step.
  – Signs of hypovolaemia include tachycardia, tachypnoea, hypotension, a postural drop in blood pressure, oliguria, confusion, cool peripheries, prolonged capillary refill time, weak thready pulse, dry mucous membranes, low JVP and reduced skin turgor.
  – Signs of hypervolaemia include peripheral oedema, hypertension, raised JVP, S3 on cardiac auscultation, bi-basal inspiratory crackles and ascites.
➤ General examination may reveal the characteristic facies and slow-relaxing ankle jerks of hypothyroidism, or the mucous membrane and skin crease pigmentation of primary adrenal insufficiency.
➤ Signs of cerebral oedema include reduced level of consciousness, fixed pupillary dilatation and seizures.
➤ Respiratory and nervous system examination may reveal evidence of chest or CNS pathology causing SIADH.

INVESTIGATIONS
➤ Paired serum and urine sodium and osmolality:
  – Serum osmolality distinguishes between hypotonic and non-hypotonic hyponatraemia.
  – The diagnosis of SIADH requires a clinically euvolaemic patient with normal hepatic, renal, cardiac, thyroid and adrenal function, who has a low serum osmolality with an inappropriately high urine osmolality (> 100 mOsm/kg) and high urine sodium (> 20 mEq/l). The increase in sodium excretion occurs in order to maintain euvolaemia in the face of water retention.
  – Primary polydipsia will result in maximally dilute urine, with a urine osmolality of < 100 mOsm/kg
  – Hypovolaemia due to renal sodium loss (e.g. due to diuretic therapy) will result in high urine sodium (> 20 mEq/l), whereas other causes of hypovolaemia will cause an appropriate avid retention of sodium by the kidneys, resulting in low urine sodium (< 20 mEq/l).
  – Hypervolaemic states such as congestive cardiac failure, nephrotic syndrome and liver cirrhosis are associated with low urine sodium (< 20 mEq/l), unless diuretics are used in treatment. Chronic renal failure is often associated with high urine sodium (>20 mEq/l), although not sufficiently high to correct the hypervolaemic state.
➤ Miscellaneous blood tests:
  – U&Es.
  – Glucose. Hyperglycaemia may cause non-hypotonic hyponatraemia.
  – Total protein and lipid profile should be checked to rule out pseudohyponatraemia.
  – LFTs and albumin levels. These may be abnormal with liver cirrhosis.
  – TFTs. Hypothyroidism is a possible cause of hyponatraemia.
  – Short tetracosactide test. This is used to diagnose adrenal insufficiency.
➤ Imaging studies:
  – CXR with or without CT of the chest should be performed in cases of SIADH, in order to diagnose an underlying pulmonary cause. CT of the head should also be performed if there is clinical evidence of intracranial pathology.

REFERENCES
1   Yeates KE, Singer M, Ross Morton A. Salt and water: a simple approach to hyponatremia. *Can Med Assoc J*. 2004; **170**: 365–9.
2   Ramrakha P, Moore K. *Oxford Handbook of Acute Medicine*. 2nd ed. Oxford: Oxford University Press; 2007. pp. 570–4.
3   Adrogue HJ, Madias NE. Hyponatremia. *NEJM*. 2000; **342**: 1581–9.

CHAPTER 35

Hypernatraemia

PATHOPHYSIOLOGY AND AETIOLOGY

Hypernatraemia may be defined as a serum sodium concentration greater than 145 mmol/l. Most cases of hypernatraemia are caused by a relative deficit of total body water causing a rise in serum osmolality and the concentration of all solutes, including sodium. A water deficit may arise as a result of reduced water consumption (e.g. in the elderly or debilitated), or due to excessive free water loss. Such water loss may occur through the renal, gastrointestinal or cutaneous routes. A person who is not incapacitated by illness or debility and who has free access to water can normally compensate for increased renal, gastrointestinal and cutaneous water losses by increasing oral water intake. However, if this is not possible, hypernatraemia may rapidly develop.

Small increases in total body sodium act mainly to expand the extracellular volume, with only minimal effects on the serum Na^+ concentration. This is because sodium is kept in the extracellular compartment by Na^+/K^+ antiporters on cell membranes. If the extracellular sodium content rises, water is drawn from the intracellular to the extracellular compartment down the resulting osmotic gradient. In addition, the increased extracellular osmolality stimulates thirst and ADH production, thus increasing total body water. However, extreme salt loading, which is usually iatrogenic, may result in significant hypernatraemia. Mineralocorticoid excess, in conditions such as Conn's syndrome or Cushing's syndrome, can result in mild hypernatraemia due to sodium retention.

The causes of hypernatraemia are listed in Table 35.1, with common causes highlighted in bold type.

EMERGENCY MANAGEMENT

Excessively rapid correction of hypernatraemia, especially if it is chronic, may be associated with cerebral oedema. The serum Na^+ concentration should therefore be corrected by no more than 10 mmol/l per day in most cases, aiming for a target of 145 mmol/l.[1] Treatment depends on the underlying cause, as described below.

Table 35.1 Causes of hypernatraemia

Water deficit	*Sodium excess*
Reduced water intake	Excessive sodium administration
	➤ Intravenous
Renal water loss	➤ Oral
➤ **Hyperosmolar non-ketotic state**	➤ Enema
➤ Nephrogenic diabetes insipidus	
➤ Cranial diabetes insipidus	Mineralocorticoid excess
➤ Renal tract obstruction (recovery)	➤ Conn's syndrome
➤ Acute tubular necrosis (recovery)	➤ Cushing's syndrome
➤ Acute interstitial nephritis	➤ Miscellaneous
➤ Tubulointerstitial disease	
➤ Diuretics	
Gastrointestinal water loss	
➤ **Diarrhoea**	
➤ **Vomiting**	
➤ Excessive stoma output	
➤ Enterocutaneous fistula	
➤ Nasogastric drainage	
Cutaneous water loss	
➤ Excessive sweating	
➤ Burns	

Replacement of water deficit

Pure water deficit is most conveniently corrected using 5% dextrose. However, if there are clinical signs of hypovolaemia that suggest concurrent sodium depletion, hypotonic saline or dextrose saline should be used. The following formula may be utilised to calculate the expected change in serum sodium concentration produced by the infusion of 1 litre of 5% dextrose, hypotonic saline or dextrose saline:[1]

$$\text{change in serum } [Na^+] = \frac{\text{infusate } [Na^+] - \text{serum } [Na^+]}{\text{total body water} + 1}$$

where total body water (l) = body weight (kg) × correction factor.

Correction factors are as follows:

non-elderly man:	0.60
non-elderly woman:	0.50
elderly man:	0.50
elderly woman:	0.45

Removal of excess sodium

In cases of hypernatraemia secondary to sodium excess, thiazide or loop diuretics may be employed to remove the excess sodium load. In severe cases, haemodialysis may be required.

Hyperosmolar non-ketotic state (HONK)

This should be treated with fluid rehydration as described above, as well as with intravenous short-acting insulin, titrated according to capillary blood glucose measurements. Common precipitating causes of HONK should be screened for and treated if present. These include sepsis and myocardial infarction.

HISTORY

➤ Polyuria, diarrhoea or vomiting and excessive sweating suggest water loss via the renal, gastrointestinal or cutaneous routes, respectively.
➤ Headache and focal neurological deficits suggest the possibility of cranial diabetes insipidus.
➤ Conditions that predispose to reduced water intake such as immobility and dementia should be noted.
➤ Drug history may include diuretics or medications that are known to cause diabetes insipidus.

EXAMINATION

➤ Assessment of the volume status helps to distinguish between water deficit (hypovolaemia or euvolaemia) and sodium excess (hypervolaemia).
  – Signs of hypovolaemia include tachycardia, tachypnoea, hypotension, a postural drop in blood pressure, oliguria, confusion, cool peripheries, prolonged capillary refill time, weak thready pulse, dry mucous membranes, low JVP and reduced skin turgor.
  – Signs of hypervolaemia include peripheral oedema, hypertension, raised JVP, S3 on cardiac auscultation, bi-basal inspiratory crackles and ascites.
➤ Urine output monitoring may reveal polyuria, suggesting renal water loss.
➤ Neurological examination may reveal bitemporal hemianopia in the presence of pituitary or hypothalamic lesions causing cranial diabetes insipidus.

INVESTIGATIONS

The following core investigations are required:
➤ Biochemistry:
  – U&Es.
  – Glucose. Severe hyperglycaemia is a feature of HONK.
  – Calcium levels. Hypercalcaemia may cause nephrogenic diabetes insipidus.
➤ Sepsis screen should be performed in cases of HONK:
  – FBC and CRP
  – blood culture
  – urine dip and MC&S
  – CXR.
➤ ECG should be performed to detect evidence of myocardial infarction, which is a possible precipitant of HONK.

The following further investigations may be required:
➤ A water deprivation test should be performed under expert supervision, and only after the serum Na+ concentration has been corrected and the acute stage of the illness has passed.

- – Water deprivation will produce a rise in serum osmolality. Failure to concentrate urine appropriately usually indicates nephrogenic or cranial diabetes insipidus.
- – A good response to exogenous vasopressin (i.e. an increase in urine osmolality) indicates cranial diabetes insipidus, whereas a poor response occurs with nephrogenic diabetes insipidus and conditions that cause an impaired medullary concentration gradient.
- ➤ Miscellaneous endocrine tests:
  - – Serum renin levels are low and aldosterone levels are raised in Conn's syndrome.
  - – The dexamethasone suppression test or a 24-hour urinary free cortisol level is used to diagnose Cushing's syndrome.
- ➤ MRI of the brain may reveal pituitary or hypothalamic lesions that are causing cranial diabetes insipidus.

REFERENCE

1   Adrogue HJ, Madias NE. Hypernatremia. *NEJM*. 2000; **342:** 1493–9.

CHAPTER 36

Hypokalaemia

PATHOPHYSIOLOGY AND AETIOLOGY

Hypokalaemia may be defined as a serum potassium concentration of less than 3.5 mmol/l. The vast majority of potassium in the body is present within the intracellular compartment, and therefore the serum potassium concentration reflects both total body potassium and the relative distribution of potassium between the intracellular and extracellular compartments.

Hypokalaemia may be caused by the following mechanisms:

1 renal potassium loss:
   ➤ mineralocorticoid excess
   ➤ excessive diuresis
   ➤ tubular disorders
   ➤ drugs
   ➤ miscellaneous
2 extra-renal electrolyte loss
3 redistribution of potassium from the extracellular to the intracellular compartment
4 poor potassium intake (rare).

With regard to the second mechanism, it should be noted that gastric contents and sweat have a relatively low potassium content, and that the hypokalaemia associated with gastric or cutaneous electrolyte loss in fact results mainly from increased renal potassium loss.[1] Loss of sodium chloride from the gastrointestinal tract or skin results in hypovolaemia with secondary hyperaldosteronism, as well as metabolic alkalosis. Both of these factors cause increased renal potassium excretion.

The causes of hypokalaemia are listed in Table 36.1, with common causes highlighted in bold type.

EMERGENCY MANAGEMENT

➤ Hypokalaemia may lead to ventricular tachycardia or fibrillation. Cardiac monitoring is therefore essential except in mild cases.
➤ Intravenous potassium replacement is essential if the serum K^+ concentration is ≤ 2.5 mmol/l, and should be strongly considered if it is ≤ 2.9 mmol/l. The rate of replacement should not normally exceed 10 mmol of potassium per hour, due to the risk of cardiac arrhythmias. However, in high-dependency settings with close cardiac monitoring, higher rates of replacement may be given for profound hypokalaemia.
➤ Mild hypokalaemia (K^+ concentration ≥ 3.0 mmol/l) can usually be treated with oral potassium supplements alone.
➤ Identify and if possible correct the underlying cause.

HISTORY

➤ Hypokalaemia is often asymptomatic, but may cause muscle weakness or polyuria.
➤ Vomiting and diarrhoea suggest gastrointestinal fluid and electrolyte loss.
➤ Take a full drug history, asking specifically about laxative or diuretic use. Note that this may be surreptitious.
➤ Ensure that the diet is adequate, and enquire specifically about liquorice intake.
➤ Note any family history of hereditary conditions that cause hypokalaemia.

EXAMINATION

➤ Blood pressure is raised in conditions of mineralocorticoid excess and in Liddle's syndrome.
➤ Assess the volume status:
   – Hypovolaemia may occur in association with excessive renal, gastrointestinal or cutaneous fluid loss, as well as with Bartter's and Gitelman's syndromes.
   – Signs of hypovolaemia include tachycardia, tachypnoea, hypotension, a postural drop in blood pressure, oliguria, confusion, cool peripheries, prolonged capillary refill time, weak thready pulse, dry mucous membranes and reduced skin turgor.
➤ General examination:
   – Chronic vomiting due to bulimia or anorexia nervosa may lead to dental caries and parotid enlargement. Additional signs of anorexia nervosa include low body mass index and lanugo hair.

Table 36.1 Causes of hypokalaemia

Renal potassium loss	Extra-renal electrolyte loss	Redistribution	Reduced intake
Mineralocorticoid excess Exogenous mineralocorticoid ➤ Corticosteroids ➤ Fludrocortisone Renin-mediated mineralocorticoid excess ➤ Renovascular disease ➤ Renal artery stenosis ➤ Renin-secreting tumour ➤ Malignant hypertension ACTH-mediated mineralocorticoid excess ➤ ACTH-producing pituitary adenoma ➤ Glucocorticoid resistance[2] ➤ Glucocorticoid-remediable aldosteronism Primary mineralocorticoid excess ➤ Conn's syndrome ➤ Cushing's disease ➤ Deoxycorticosterone-secreting tumour ➤ 11-β-hydroxylase deficiency ➤ 17-α-hydroxylase deficiency 11-β-hydroxysteroid dehydrogenase type 2 inactivity ➤ Syndrome of apparent mineralocorticoid excess ➤ Carbenoxolone ➤ Chewing tobacco ➤ Liquorice excess Activating mineralocorticoid receptor mutation[3] *Miscellaneous* Excessive diuresis ➤ Diuretics ➤ Diabetic ketoacidosis ➤ Hyperosmolar non-ketotic state ➤ Miscellaneous Tubular disorders ➤ Bartter's syndrome ➤ Liddle's syndrome ➤ Gitelman's syndrome ➤ Type 1 or type 2 renal tubular acidosis Drugs and toxins ➤ Carbonic anhydrase inhibitors ➤ Penicillins ➤ Aminoglycosides ➤ Amphotericin B ➤ Cisplatin ➤ Toluene Miscellaneous ➤ Metabolic alkalosis ➤ Hypomagnesaemia	Gastrointestinal ➤ Vomiting ➤ Nasogastric suction ➤ Diarrhoea ➤ Laxative abuse ➤ Villous adenoma ➤ Congenital chloridorrhoea ➤ Miscellaneous Cutaneous ➤ Cystic fibrosis ➤ Excessive sweating	Drugs and toxins ➤ β2 agonists ➤ Insulin ➤ Theophylline ➤ Miscellaneous Rapid cell division ➤ Acute leukaemia[4] ➤ Lymphoma ➤ Vitamin B_{12} replacement ➤ GM-CSF Miscellaneous ➤ Alkalaemia ➤ Refeeding syndrome ➤ Hypokalaemic periodic paralysis	Malnutrition Total parenteral nutrition

- Signs of Cushing's syndrome include centripetal obesity, buffalo hump, moon face, abdominal striae, plethora and proximal muscle wasting.
➤ Abdominal examination may reveal a flank mass representing a renin-secreting renal-cell carcinoma or an abdominal bruit due to renal artery stenosis.

INVESTIGATIONS
The following core investigations are required:
➤ ECG may show characteristic changes of hypokalaemia, including prominent U waves and small P waves.
➤ Blood tests:
- U&Es.
- Magnesium levels. Hypomagnesaemia may cause hypokalaemia that is refractory to treatment.
- Phosphate levels. These fall as part of the refeeding syndrome.
- Glucose. Hyperglycaemia may cause an osmotic diuresis with potassium wasting.

The following further investigations may be required:
➤ Arterial blood gas:
- Metabolic alkalosis may occur with severe hypokalaemia in general, and particularly with conditions of mineralocorticoid excess, as well as in Bartter's, Liddle's and Gitelman's syndromes.
- Metabolic acidosis may occur in association with diarrhoea, renal tubular acidosis and carbonic anhydrase inhibitor use.
➤ Endocrine tests:
- The dexamethasone suppression test and 24-hour urinary free cortisol level are used to diagnose Cushing's syndrome.
- Plasma renin and aldosterone levels may be helpful for distinguishing between the various causes of mineralocorticoid excess. For example, Conn's syndrome causes low renin and high aldosterone levels, whereas renovascular disease causes elevated levels of both renin and aldosterone.
➤ Urinary K$^+$ excretion of < 20 mEq/24 hours indicates appropriate renal conservation, whereas a value of > 20 mEq/24 hours suggests renal potassium wasting.[1]
➤ Urinary diuretic and laxative screen.
➤ USS, CT or MR angiography may reveal renal artery stenosis or a hormone-secreting renal or adrenal tumour.

REFERENCES
1   Weiner ID, Wingo CS. Hypokalemia – consequences, causes and correction. *J Am Soc Nephrol.* 1997; **8**: 1179–88.
2   Charmandari E, Kino T, Ichijo T *et al.* Generalized glucocorticoid resistance: clinical aspects, molecular mechanisms and implications of a rare genetic disorder. *J Clin Endocrinol Metab.* 2008; **93**: 1563–72.
3   Geller DS, Farhi A, Pinkerton N *et al.* Activating mineralocorticoid receptor mutation in hypertension exacerbated by pregnancy. *Science.* 2000; **289**: 119–23.
4   Milionis HJ, Bourantas CL, Siamopoulos KC *et al.* Acid–base and electrolyte abnormalities in patients with acute leukaemia. *Am J Haematol.* 1999; **62**: 201–7.

CHAPTER 37

Hyperkalaemia

PATHOPHYSIOLOGY AND AETIOLOGY

Hyperkalaemia may be defined as a serum potassium concentration greater than 5.0 mmol/l. Since the vast majority of potassium is stored in the intracellular compartment, hyperkalaemia may reflect the redistribution of potassium into the extracellular space, rather than increased total body potassium. In some cases (e.g. in diabetic ketoacidosis), total body potassium may even be low.

The mechanisms of hyperkalaemia are as follows:

1 excessive potassium intake
2 inadequate renal potassium excretion
3 redistribution of potassium from the intracellular to the extracellular space.

A number of factors may cause a falsely high measured K^+ concentration. This is known as pseudohyperkalaemia.

The causes of hyperkalaemia are listed in Table 37.1, with common causes highlighted in bold type.

EMERGENCY MANAGEMENT

Severe hyperkalaemia must be corrected as a matter of urgency, due to its potential to cause life-threatening cardiac arrhythmias, culminating in asystole. The danger is more pronounced when potassium levels rise acutely.

The treatment priorities are as follows:

1 Protect against cardiac arrhythmias.
   ➤ If hyperkalaemic ECG changes are present, and in any case if the serum potassium concentration is greater than 6.5 mmol/l, calcium gluconate 10%, 10 ml over 10 minutes, should be administered intravenously. This may be repeated if ECG changes do not resolve.
   ➤ Cardiac monitoring should be instituted.

Table 37.1 Causes of hyperkalaemia

Excessive intake	Inadequate renal excretion	Redistribution	Pseudohyperkalaemia
Oral or intravenous potassium supplements	Renal failure	Diabetic ketoacidosis	Haemolysed sample
High-potassium diet	Hyporeninaemic hypoaldosteronism	Hyperosmolar non-ketotic state	Tight tourniquet
			Leukocytosis
Upper gastrointestinal haemorrhage	Drugs	Acidaemia	
	➤ Potassium-sparing diuretics		Thrombocytosis
		Cell lysis	
Blood transfusion	➤ ACE inhibitors	➤ Rhabdomyolysis	
	➤ Angiotensin II receptor antagonists	➤ Tumour lysis syndrome	
		➤ Malignant hyperpyrexia	
	➤ NSAIDs	➤ Massive haemolysis	
	➤ Miscellaneous	➤ Burns	
		➤ Exercise	
	Adrenal insufficiency		
		Hyperkalaemic periodic paralysis	
	Pseudohypoaldosteronism		
	Mineralocorticoid synthetic defects	Drugs and toxins	
		➤ Beta-blockers	
	➤ 21-Hydroxylase deficiency	➤ Digoxin	
		➤ Succinylcholine	
	➤ Aldosterone synthase deficiency	➤ Miscellaneous	

2   Lower the serum potassium concentration.
  ➤ Insulin acts to redistribute extracellular potassium into the intracellular space. An intravenous infusion of 10 units of rapid-acting insulin in 50 ml of 50% dextrose given over 30 minutes will lower the serum potassium concentration with approximately neutral effects on blood glucose (first-line therapy).
  ➤ Nebulised salbutamol acts to shift potassium into the intracellular compartment, due to its β-agonist effects.
  ➤ Correction of metabolic acidosis, if present, with IV sodium bicarbonate may also serve to lower the serum potassium concentration by causing redistribution of potassium into the intracellular compartment.
  ➤ Severe refractory hyperkalaemia may require dialysis for correction, particularly in patients with severe renal impairment.
  ➤ Ion-exchange resins such as calcium resonium increase potassium excretion via the gastrointestinal tract. These do not lower potassium acutely, but act over a period of hours or days, helping to keep potassium levels down once the treatment described above has been instituted.
3   Stop medications that may raise the serum potassium concentration.
4   Institute a low-potassium diet.

HISTORY
➤ Symptoms of hyperkalaemia are non-specific and include muscle weakness and fatigue.
➤ Oliguria or anuria may herald acute kidney injury.
➤ Drug history. Potassium-sparing diuretics, ACE inhibitors, angiotensin-II receptor antagonists and NSAIDs are common causes of hyperkalaemia.
➤ Enquire about the patient's intake of high-potassium foods, such as fruit, vegetables, fruit juice and low-sodium salts.

EXAMINATION
➤ Signs of hyperkalaemia include bradycardia and generalised muscle weakness.
➤ Mucous membrane or skin crease pigmentation suggests primary adrenal insufficiency.
➤ Check carefully for a palpable bladder, which indicates urinary outflow tract obstruction. This is an easily correctable cause of acute kidney injury and thus hyperkalaemia.

INVESTIGATIONS
The following core investigations are required:
➤ ECG may show a number of characteristic changes. The following changes mandate urgent treatment, as they may herald deterioration to asystole:
  – peaked T waves
  – widened QRS complexes
  – prolonged PR interval and small P waves
  – sine wave pattern (pre-arrest).
➤ Blood tests:
    U&Es may reveal renal impairment. Hyponatraemia occurs with mineralocorticoid deficiency or resistance.
  – FBC may reveal evidence of upper gastrointestinal haemorrhage or haemolysis, which are both possible causes of hyperkalaemia.
  – Glucose is raised with diabetic ketoacidosis and hyperosmolar non-ketotic state.

The following further investigations may be required:
➤ Creatine kinase activity. This is raised with rhabdomyolysis, malignant hyperpyrexia, vigorous exercise and burns.
➤ Uric acid levels. These are raised with tumour lysis syndrome.
➤ Short tetracosactide test. This may be diagnostic of primary adrenal insufficiency.

CHAPTER 38

Hypocalcaemia

PATHOPHYSIOLOGY AND AETIOLOGY

Under normal circumstances, approximately 50% of serum calcium is protein-bound and 50% is in the physiologically active ionised form. Hypoalbuminaemia increases the proportion of calcium that is ionised, whereas hyperalbuminaemia reduces this proportion. Since most laboratories measure total rather than ionised calcium, it is conventional to apply a correction factor to the serum calcium concentration ($[Ca^{2+}]$) in order to obtain a better measure of physiologically active serum calcium levels. The following formula is commonly used, with serum albumin concentration ([albumin]) measured in g/l:

$$\text{corrected } [Ca^{2+}] = \text{uncorrected } [Ca^{2+}] + 0.02 \times (40 - \text{serum [albumin]}).$$

Acidaemia increases the proportion of calcium that is ionised, whereas alkalaemia has the opposite effect. Thus acute respiratory alkalosis (e.g. due to a panic attack) may cause hypocalcaemic tetany as a result of a reduction in ionised calcium levels. However, the total serum calcium level remains unchanged.

Hypocalcaemia may be defined as a corrected serum calcium concentration of < 2.2 mmol/l. It may be caused by the following mechanisms:

1 vitamin D deficiency or resistance
2 parathyroid hormone (PTH) deficiency or resistance
3 calcium sequestration
4 excessive renal calcium excretion
5 reduced gastrointestinal calcium absorption.

The causes of hypocalcaemia are shown in Table 38.1, with common causes highlighted in bold type.

Table 38.1 Causes of hypocalcaemia[1]

Vitamin D deficiency or resistance	Parathyroid hormone deficiency or resistance	Calcium sequestration	Miscellaneous
Inadequate dietary intake	Parathyroid trauma ➤ **Parathyroidectomy** ➤ **Thyroidectomy** ➤ Neck irradiation	Acute pancreatitis	Excessive renal calcium excretion ➤ **Loop diuretics** ➤ Fanconi syndrome
Malabsorption		Hyperphosphataemia	
Inadequate sunlight exposure	Neoplasia ➤ Parathyroid cancer ➤ Thyroid cancer ➤ Metastases	Bone calcium uptake ➤ Osteoblastic metastases ➤ **Hungry bone syndrome** ➤ Bisphosphonates ➤ Oestrogens	Reduced gastrointestinal calcium absorption ➤ Proton pump inhibitors ➤ H$_2$ receptor antagonists
Renal failure			
Hepatic failure	Hypomagnesaemia		Toxic shock syndrome
Oncogenic osteomalacia	Autoimmune	Cell lysis ➤ Rhabdomyolysis ➤ Tumour lysis syndrome	
Familial ➤ X-linked hypophosphataemia ➤ 1α-Hydroxylase deficiency	Infiltration ➤ Thalassaemia major ➤ Haemochromatosis ➤ Wilson's disease ➤ Sarcoidosis ➤ Amyloidosis	Drugs and toxins ➤ Foscarnet ➤ Blood transfusion ➤ Ethylene glycol ➤ Miscellaneous	
Drugs ➤ Phenobarbital ➤ Phenytoin ➤ Miscellaneous	Hereditary ➤ PTH deficiency ➤ PTH resistance		
	Drugs and toxins ➤ Cinacalcet ➤ Alcohol		

EMERGENCY MANAGEMENT
➤ Severe hypocalcaemia may cause seizures or cardiac arrhythmias.
➤ Mild hypocalcaemia should be treated with oral calcium/vitamin D supplements, whereas severe hypocalcaemia requires intravenous calcium replacement.

HISTORY
➤ Symptoms of hypocalcaemia include paraesthesiae, muscle cramps or tetany, carpopedal spasm, dysphagia, dysphonia, wheeze and seizures.
➤ Family history of inherited hypocalcaemic conditions should be noted.
➤ Take a dietary history. Asian women living in temperate areas are particularly at risk of vitamin D deficiency, due to their lack of adequate dietary intake or sunlight exposure.

EXAMINATION
➤ Check for signs of cardiac failure, which is a possible consequence of hypocalcaemia. Clinical features may include crackles at the lung bases, raised JVP, S3 gallop rhythm and peripheral oedema.
➤ Chvostek's sign is contraction of the ipsilateral facial muscles upon tapping the facial nerve as it passes in front of the ear. It is a sign of neuromuscular excitability that is seen with hypocalcaemia.
➤ Trousseau's sign is carpopedal spasm elicited by inflation of a sphygmomanometer cuff around the arm. It is a further sign of neuromuscular excitability.
➤ Involuntary movements due to basal ganglia calcification occur in some cases of chronic hypocalcaemia due to hypoparathyroidism or parathyroid hormone resistance.

INVESTIGATIONS
➤ ECG may reveal a prolonged QT interval.
➤ Blood tests:
   – U&Es and LFTs. Renal failure and less commonly liver cirrhosis may cause reduced metabolism of vitamin D to its active form, resulting in hypocalcaemia.
   – ALP activity. This may be low with PTH deficiency and raised with vitamin D deficiency.
   – Phosphate levels. These are raised with renal failure and PTH deficiency, and low with vitamin D deficiency and conditions of increased bone calcium uptake.
   – Magnesium levels. Hypomagnesaemia depresses PTH release.
   – Vitamin D levels. Deficiency is a common cause of hypocalcaemia.
   – PTH levels. These are low with PTH deficiency and raised with PTH resistance.
   – Amylase activity is raised with acute pancreatitis.

REFERENCE
1   Thakker RV. Parathyroid disorders and diseases altering calcium metabolism. In: Warrell DA, Cox TM, Firth JD (eds) *Oxford Textbook of Medicine*. 4th ed. Oxford: Oxford University Press; 2003. pp. 2.230–2.241.

CHAPTER 39

Hypercalcaemia

PATHOPHYSIOLOGY AND AETIOLOGY

Hypercalcaemia may be defined as a corrected serum calcium concentration ($[Ca^{2+}]$) greater than 2.6 mmol/l, where:

$$corrected\ [Ca^{2+}] = uncorrected\ [Ca^{2+}] + 0.02 \times (40 - serum\ [albumin]).$$

The correction for albumin is necessary because a reduction in serum albumin concentration (measured in g/l) increases the fraction of calcium that is ionised and hence physiologically active, and vice versa.

Hypercalcaemia may be caused by the following mechanisms:
1 excess vitamin D
2 excess PTH or PTH-related peptide
3 increased calcium resorption from bone
4 reduced renal calcium excretion
5 excessive calcium intake
6 miscellaneous mechanisms.

The causes of hypercalcaemia are listed in Table 39.1, with common causes highlighted in bold type.

EMERGENCY MANAGEMENT

➤ Intravenous rehydration with normal saline (e.g. 4 litres over 24 hours).
➤ Additional treatment is dependent on the underlying cause. For instance, malignant hypercalcaemia is treated with IV pamidronate, whereas hypercalcaemia due to sarcoidosis requires corticosteroids.

HISTORY

➤ Symptoms of hypercalcaemia include abdominal pain, nausea, vomiting, constipation, polyuria, depression, confusion and myalgia.
➤ Associated symptoms:
  – Haematuria or loin pain suggests renal calculi, which are a possible consequence of hypercalcaemia.
  – Fever, night sweats and weight loss may occur with lymphoma.
  – Dyspnoea or cough suggests granulomatous lung disease or lung cancer.
  – Bone pain may occur with multiple myeloma or other malignant bone infiltrations.
➤ Drug history. Note in particular any use of thiazide diuretics or calcium-containing indigestion remedies.
➤ Family history may reveal a hereditary condition that predisposes to hypercalcaemia.

EXAMINATION

➤ Check for signs of hypovolaemia, as hypercalcaemia may cause polyuria and excessive renal fluid loss.
➤ Lymphadenopathy occurs with lymphoma and metastatic malignancy.
➤ Chest examination may reveal signs of lung cancer or granulomatous lung disease.
➤ Abdominal examination may reveal hepatomegaly due to metastatic malignancy, or splenomegaly due to lymphoma.

INVESTIGATIONS

➤ ECG may reveal a shortened QT interval.
➤ Biochemistry and immunology:
  – U&Es may show renal impairment.
  – Phosphate levels are low or normal with PTH or PTH-related peptide excess, and raised with vitamin D excess.
  – ALP activity is raised in conditions of excess bone resorption.
  – PTH levels are raised in primary and tertiary hyperparathyroidism.
  – Vitamin D levels.
  – TFTs may reveal hyperthyroidism.
  – Serum ACE activity is often raised in sarcoidosis.
  – Serum electrophoresis, serum free light chains and urinary Bence Jones protein are used to diagnose multiple myeloma.

Table 39.1 Causes of hypercalcaemia[1,2]

Vitamin D excess	PTH or PTH-related peptide excess	Increased bone resorption	Reduced renal excretion	Excessive calcium intake	Miscellaneous
Granulomatous disease	Parathyroid adenoma	Multiple myeloma	Thiazide diuretics	Milk-alkali syndrome	Mixed or unclear mechanism
➤ Sarcoidosis	Parathyroid hyperplasia	Bone metastases	Familial hypocalciuric hypercalcaemia	Calcium carbonate ingestion	➤ Rhabdomyolysis (recovery)
➤ Berylliosis	Parathyroid cancer	Primary bone tumour		Total parenteral nutrition	➤ Chronic liver disease
➤ Tuberculosis	Tertiary hyperparathyroidism	Adynamic bone disease			➤ Adrenal insufficiency
➤ Leprosy	Humoral hypercalcaemia of malignancy	Hyperthyroidism			➤ VIPoma
➤ Coccidioidomycosis	Ectopic PTH secretion	Drugs			Pseudohypercalcaemia
➤ Histoplasmosis	Phaeochromocytoma	➤ Vitamin A toxicity			➤ Tourniquet
➤ Miscellaneous	Lithium	➤ Oestrogens			➤ Paraproteinaemia
Lymphoma	Theophylline	➤ Oestrogen antagonists			
Vitamin D toxicity		➤ Testosterone			
		➤ Miscellaneous			

- – The urinary calcium/creatinine clearance ratio is low in familial hypocalciuric hypercalcaemia.
➤ Imaging:
  - – CXR may show bilateral hilar lymphadenopathy (which suggests sarcoidosis, lymphoma or tuberculosis), lung cancer or granulomatous lung disease.
  - – Skeletal survey or isotope bone scan may reveal evidence of multiple myeloma, bone metastases or a primary bone tumour.

REFERENCES

1 Thakker RV. Parathyroid disorders and diseases altering calcium metabolism. In: Warrell DA, Cox TM, Firth JD (eds) *Oxford Textbook of Medicine*. 4th ed. Oxford: Oxford University Press; 2003. pp. 2.230–2.241.
2 Jacobs TP, Bilezikian JP. Rare causes of hypercalcemia. *J Clin Endocrinol Metab*. 2005; **90**: 6316–22.

Index

AACG *see* acute angle-closure glaucoma
ABCD (airway, breathing, circulation, disability) 7–9
abdominal aortic aneurysm
  abdominal pain 51, 54
  anaemia 124
  back pain 114
  shock 20
abdominal pain 51–6
  back pain 117
  emergency management 51
  examination 54–5
  history 51, 54
  investigations 55–6
  pathophysiology and aetiology 51, 52–3
abdominal swelling 74–6
abdominal wall tenderness test 55
abnormally forceful cardiac contraction 41
abnormal pulse rate or rhythm 41
absolute constipation 72
acidaemia 152
acid–base disturbances 133–9
  compensatory responses 134
  metabolic acidosis 134–7
  metabolic alkalosis 138, 139
  respiratory acid–base disturbances 134–5, 136
  standard base excess 133–4
acidosis 16, 17, 133, 134–7
acute angle-closure glaucoma (AACG) 83, 86, 98, 99
acute haemorrhage 18, 124, 127
acute interstitial nephritis 27, 28–9
acute kidney injury (AKI) 27–31
acute limb ischaemia 49
acute monoarthritis 110
acute respiratory acidosis 134
acute respiratory alkalosis 134, 152
acute respiratory illness 10–17
  emergency management 13–15
  examination 16
  history 15–16
  investigations 16–17
  pathophysiology and aetiology 10–13
acute tubular necrosis 27, 28–9
acute visual loss 98–100
ADH (antidiuretic hormone) 103, 140–4
advanced cardiac resuscitation 7
airflow limitation 15
airway
  acute respiratory illness 13
  anaemia 124
  coma and reduced level of consciousness 22
  critically ill patient 7–8
  dysphagia 65
  gastrointestinal haemorrhage 62, 64
  nausea and vomiting 57
AKI *see* acute kidney injury
alcohol
  abdominal pain 54
  abdominal swelling 74
  coma and reduced level of consciousness 22, 25
  gastrointestinal haemorrhage 64
  palpitation – history 44

alkalaemia 152
alkalosis 133, 134, 138, 139, 147, 152
alveolar–arterial gradient (A–a gradient) 16–17, 35
alveolar ventilation 10, 16
amaurosis fugax 98, 100
amoebic dysentery 64
anaemia 124–8
  abdominal pain 54
  acute respiratory illness 17
  diarrhoea 71
  emergency management 124
  examination 127
  gastrointestinal haemorrhage 62
  haematuria 107
  history 124, 127
  investigations 127–8
  pathophysiology and aetiology 124, 125–6
anal fissures 73
anaphylaxis
  acute respiratory illness 15
  dysphagia 65
  shock 18, 20
  skin rash 129
angina 37
angioedema 65, 129
anion gap (AG) 136, 137
anorexia nervosa 139, 147
antidiuretic hormone (ADH) 103, 141, 144
aortic dissection
  abdominal pain 55
  back pain 114, 117
  non-pleuritic chest pain 37, 39, 40
  shock 18, 20
aortic regurgitation 44
appendicitis 51, 55
arrhythmias *see* cardiac arrhythmias
arterial blood gas analysis 16–17, 91
arterial occlusion 49
arthritis 110, 117
ascites 55, 74, 75, 80
asthma 15
asystole 150
ataxia 57, 91, 95
availability bias 5

back pain 114–18
bacterial dysentery 64
bacterial meningitis 22
bacterial pneumonia 33
bandwagon effect 5
barbiturates 16
Bartter's syndrome 147
basal ganglia 91, 153
base rate neglect 5
Behçet's disease 110, 122
benzodiazepines 16
bias 5
bilious vomiting 57
bilirubin 77
biochemical abnormalities 133–56
  acid–base disturbances 133–9
  hypercalcaemia 154–6
  hyperkalaemia 150–1
  hypernatraemia 144–6
  hypocalcaemia 152–3
  hypokalaemia 147–9
  hyponatraemia 140–3
bitemporal hemianopia 145

blood pressure
  acute visual loss 98
  critically ill patient 9
  non-pleuritic chest pain 39
  palpitation 41, 43, 44
  shock 20
blood tests 1
Boerhaave's syndrome 37
bone-marrow failure 124
Bouchard's nodes 113
Boutonnière deformity 113
bowel dilatation 74
bowel obstruction
  abdominal pain 54, 55
  abdominal swelling 74
  constipation 72, 73
  nausea and vomiting 57, 60
bradyarrhythmias 18, 43, 44
brain
  coma and reduced level of consciousness 22
  focal neurological deficit 91, 92, 95
breast cancer 35, 122
breathing 8–9, 62, 64, 124
British Thoracic Society 35
Brudzinski's sign 86
Buerger's test 49
bulbar palsy 65, 67
bulimia 139, 147

caffeine 44
calcium
  hypercalcaemia 154–6
  hypocalcaemia 152–3
carbon monoxide poisoning 88, 89
cardiac arrhythmias
  hypocalcaemia 153
  hypokalaemia 147
  non-pleuritic chest pain 39
  palpitation 41, 43, 44
  pseudohyperkalaemia 150
  shock 18, 20
  transient loss of consciousness 88
cardiac ischaemia 41
cardiac murmurs 20
cardiac tamponade 18, 20, 34
cardiac wheeze 15
cardiogenic shock 18, 19, 20
cardiorespiratory arrest (cardiac arrest) 7, 8
cardiovascular and respiratory presentations 33–50
  limb pain 49–50
  non-pleuritic chest pain 37–40
  oedema 45–8
  palpitation 41–4
  pleuritic chest pain 33–6
cauda equina syndrome
  back pain 114, 117
  constipation 72, 73
  focal neurological deficit 91, 95, 96
cellulitis 49
central pontine myelinolysis (CPN) 141
cerebellar disease 91, 94, 96
cerebral oedema 140, 141, 143, 144
chest pain 6, 44, 57 *see also* non-pleuritic chest pain; pleuritic chest pain
cholangitis 77
cholecystitis 77

chronic liver disease 77, 80
chronic obstructive pulmonary disease (COPD) 9, 13, 15, 34, 46
chronic respiratory acidosis 134
chronic respiratory alkalosis 134
Chvostek's sign 153
circulation 9, 62, 64, 124
Clostridium difficile 68
clubbing 16, 71
cocaine 39
coeliac disease 71
coffee-ground vomiting 20, 57, 62, 127
cognitive errors in diagnosis 5
colectomy 68
coma and reduced level of consciousness 22–6
compartment syndrome 49
confirmation bias 5
confusion in the elderly 22, 23
congestive cardiac failure 34, 41, 143
Conn's syndrome 144, 146
consciousness
    acute respiratory illness 16
    coma and reduced level of consciousness 22–6
    critically ill patient 9
    transient loss of consciousness 88–90
constant positive airway pressure (CPAP) 15
constipation 54, 72–3, 127
constrictive pericarditis 80
contingency tables 2
COPD see chronic obstructive pulmonary disease
coronary heart disease 39
cor pulmonale 16, 46
cough
    acute respiratory illness 10, 13, 14
    anaemia 127
    hypercalcaemia 154
    hyponatraemia 141
    non-pleuritic chest pain 39
    pleuritic chest pain 34
Courvoisier's sign 80
cranial diabetes insipidus
    frequency of micturition 103, 104, 106
    hypernatraemia 145, 146
cranial nerves 65, 95
critical illness 7–31
    acute kidney injury 27–31
    acute respiratory illness 10–17
    coma and reduced level of consciousness 22–6
    critically ill patient 7–9
    shock 18–21
Crohn's disease 71, 110, 122
crystal arthropathies 110
Cullen's sign 55
Curriculum for General Internal Medicine vi
Cushing's syndrome 139, 144, 146, 149
cystitis 105

D-dimer 2, 3, 35
deep vein thrombosis 34, 35, 46, 49
dementia 145
diabetes 100, 103, 104, 145, 146
diabetic ketoacidosis
    abdominal pain 54
    acute respiratory illness 16, 17
    coma and reduced level of consciousness 25
    frequency of micturition 103, 105
    hyperkalaemia 150
    nausea and vomiting 57

diagnostic tests 1–3
diagnostic thinking 4–6
    cognitive errors in diagnosis 5
    diagnosis by exhaustion 4
    diagnosis in clinical practice 5–6
    diagnostic error 4–5
    diagnostic strategies 4
    pathological sieve 4
diarrhoea 68–71
    abdominal pain 54
    anaemia 127
    emergency management 68
    examination 68, 71
    history 68
    investigations 71
    joint pain or swelling 110
    nausea and vomiting 57
    pathophysiology and aetiology 68, 69–70
diet 57, 68, 73, 140, 153
differential diagnosis 1
dilutional acidosis 136
disability 9
distributive shock 18, 19
Doppler scan 35, 48, 50
driving 88
drug history 1
drug misuse see illicit drug use
dysarthria 95
dysentery 64
dysphagia 65–7, 127
dysphasia 95
dyspnoea
    acute respiratory illness 10, 13, 15, 16
    dysphagia 65
    hypercalcaemia 154
    hyponatraemia 141
    non-pleuritic chest pain 39
    pleuritic chest pain 34

ecstasy 143
ectopic pregnancy 51, 54, 124
eczema herpeticum 129
effective arterial blood volume (EABV) 140
elderly people 22, 23, 140
emphysema 80
empyema 33, 55
endotracheal intubation 8
epididymo-orchitis 107
epiglottitis 65
errors 4–5
erythroderma 129
euvolaemia 140, 141, 142, 143, 145
examination 1, 4
extracranial disease 83, 84–5
extrahepatic cholestasis 77, 78–9, 80
extrapyramidal disease 91, 94, 95
eyes 95, 98–100

faeculent vomiting 57
family history 1
faulty context generation 5
faulty data interpretation 5
faulty triggering 5
fixed acids 133
focal neurological deficit 91–7
    acute visual loss 99
    emergency management 91
    examination 95–6
    history 91, 95
    investigations 96–7
    pathophysiology and aetiology 91, 92, 93
food poisoning 57
forced vital capacity (FVC) 91

frequency of micturition 103–6
    emergency management 103, 105
    examination 105
    history 105
    investigations 105–6
    pathophysiology and aetiology 103, 104
fulminant hepatic failure 77, 80

gait 95
gallstone disease 77
gastrointestinal haemorrhage 62–4
gastrointestinal presentations 51–81
    abdominal pain 51–6
    abdominal swelling 74–6
    constipation 72–3
    diarrhoea 68–71
    dysphagia 65–7
    gastrointestinal haemorrhage 62–4
    jaundice 77–81
    nausea and vomiting 57–61
GCS see Glasgow Coma Scale
generalised oedema 45, 46, 47
generalised pustular psoriasis 129
Geneva score 35
genitalia 55
giant-cell arteritis 83, 86, 98, 100
Giardia lamblia 68
Gitelman's syndrome 147
Glasgow Coma Scale (GCS) 7, 9, 16, 22, 25, 86
global cerebral dysfunction 22
glomerular disease 27, 28–9
glomerulonephritis 46
goitre 119
gonorrhoea 68
Goodpasture's disease 17
Grey–Turner's sign 55
Guillain–Barré syndrome 16, 117

haematemesis 20, 62, 127
haematuria 46, 107–9, 127
haemodialysis 145
haemoglobin 124
haemolysis 125–6
haemoptysis 15
Hallpike test 101
headache 83–7
    emergency management 83
    examination 86
    history 83
    investigations 86–7
    nausea and vomiting 57
    pathophysiology and aetiology 83, 84–5
Heberden's nodes 113
hemiplegia 95
Henderson equation 133, 135
heparin 49
hepatic flap 57
hepatitis 74, 77
hepatomegaly 74, 77, 154
hernia 55, 74
heroin 16
heuristics 5
history 1, 4
HIV (human immunodeficiency virus) 119
HONK see hyperosmolar non-ketotic state
hyperalbuminaemia 136
hyperaldosteronism 147
hyperbilirubinaemia 77
hypercalcaemia 154–6
hypercapnia 14, 16
hypercapnic (type 2) respiratory failure 10–13, 15

hyperchloraemic acidosis *see* metabolic acidosis
hyperglycaemia 100, 140
hyperkalaemia 27, 150–1
hypernatraemia 103, 105, 144–6
hyperosmolar non-ketotic state (HONK) 103, 145
hypertension 44, 98, 139
hyperthyroidism 41, 44
hypertrophic cardiomyopathy 88
hyperventilation 134
hypervolaemia 140, 141, 142, 143, 145
hypoalbuminaemia
 abdominal swelling 74
 acid–base disturbances 136, 139
 hypocalcaemia 152
 oedema 45, 46
hypocalcaemia 152–3
hypoglycaemia 9, 22, 41, 88
hypokalaemia 27, 147–9
hyponatraemia 140–3
hypotension 20, 41, 43, 44
hypothalamus 119
hypothetico-deductive method 4
hypothyroidism 140
hypotonic hyponatraemia 140, 142, 143
hypoventilation 134
hypovolaemia
 abdominal pain 54
 acid–base disturbances 139
 acute kidney injury 27, 30
 anaemia 127
 diarrhoea 68
 frequency of micturition 103, 105
 gastrointestinal haemorrhage 62, 64
 haematuria 107
 hypercalcaemia 154
 hypernatraemia 145
 hypokalaemia 147
 hyponatraemia 140, 141, 142, 143
 nausea and vomiting 57
 shock 18, 19, 20
 transient loss of consciousness 89
hypoxaemic (type 1) respiratory failure 10–12, 15
hypoxia 13, 14, 16, 88

illicit drug use 16, 39, 44, 143
'illness script' 1
impaired diffusion 10
infective endocarditis 119, 127, 132
inflammatory arthritis 110, 117
inflammatory bowel disease 68, 71
information gathering and interpretation 1–3
insulin 103, 105
interpretation of test results 1 3
interstitial fluid 45
intracranial disease 83, 84–5
intrinsic liver disease 77, 78–9
investigations 1, 4, 6
iron-deficiency anaemia 5–6
ischaemic heart disease 20
ischaemic stroke 91, 100

jaundice 77–81
 abdominal pain 54
 abdominal swelling 74
 anaemia 127
 emergency management 77
 examination 77, 80
 history 77
 investigations 80–1
 nausea and vomiting 57
 pathophysiology and aetiology 77, 78–9
 pyrexia of unknown origin 119

jaw thrust 7
joint pain or swelling 110–13
jugular venous pressure (JVP)
 abdominal swelling 75
 jaundice 80
 non-pleuritic chest pain 39
 oedema 46
 pleuritic chest pain 34
 shock 20
 transient loss of consciousness 89

Kayser–Fleischer rings 80
keratitis 98
Kernig's sign 86
ketoacidosis 135
kidneys
 acid–base disturbances 134
 acute kidney injury 27–31
 frequency of micturition 103
 hyponatraemia 140
Kussmaul's sign 46, 75, 80
kyphosis 117

lactic acidosis 135
laryngeal mask 8
Liddle's syndrome 139, 147
limb pain 49–50
liver cirrhosis 74, 140, 143
liver transplantation 77
local infection 23–4
localised oedema 45, 46, 47
lower motor neuron lesions 91, 96
lung cancer 127, 154
lymphadenopathy 54, 119, 154
lymphatic system 45, 46
lymphoma 154
lymphoscintigraphy 48

macrocytic anaemia 124, 125–6
malignant bone infiltration 49
malignant hyperpyrexia 91
mean corpuscular volume (MCV) 124
mechanical bowel obstruction 72, 73
medical diagnosis
 diagnostic thinking 4–6
 information gathering and interpretation 1–3
melaena
 anaemia 127
 gastrointestinal haemorrhage 62
 nausea and vomiting 57, 60
 shock 20
meningitis 25, 83, 86
meningococcal sepsis 129
menorrhagia 127
menstruation 54
metabolic acid–base disturbances 16–17, 133–9, 147
metabolic acidosis 16, 17, 134–7
metabolic alkalosis 134, 138, 139, 147
microcytic anaemia 124, 125–6
micturition *see* frequency of micturition
migraine 83
miscellaneous presentations 103–32
 anaemia 124–8
 back pain 114–18
 frequency of micturition 103–6
 haematuria 107–9
 joint pain or swelling 110–13
 pyrexia of unknown origin 119–23
 skin rash 129–32
monoarthritis 110
movement abnormalities 91, 94
Murphy's sign 55
myelopathy 91
myocardial infarction 18, 20, 88

myocardial ischaemia 39

nausea and vomiting 57–61
 abdominal pain 54
 acid–base disturbances 139
 airway 7
 emergency management 57
 examination 57, 60
 gastrointestinal haemorrhage 62
 history 57
 hypokalaemia 147
 investigations 60
 non-pleuritic chest pain 39
 pathophysiology and aetiology 58–9
necrotising fasciitis 49, 129
negative predictive value (NPV) 2, 3, 5
nephrogenic diabetes insipidus 103, 104, 146
nephrotic syndrome 140, 143
nerve root damage 91, 96, 117
nervous system 114
neurogenic claudication 49
neurological presentations 83–102
 acute visual loss 98–100
 focal neurological deficit 91–7
 headache 83–7
 transient loss of consciousness 88–90
 vertigo 101–2
neuromuscular dysfunction 91, 93
neuromuscular dysphagia 65
neuromyotonia 91
neuropathic pain 33, 51, 54
neutropenia 119
nigrostriatal pathway 91
non hypotonic hyponatraemia 140–1, 142, 143
non-pleuritic chest pain 37–40
non-ST elevation myocardial infarction (NSTEMI) 37
normocytic anaemia 124, 125–6
NPV (negative predictive value) 2, 3, 5
nystagmus 25, 101

obesity 16, 74
obstructive shock 18, 19
obstructive sleep apnoea 13, 16
obturator sign 55
oedema 45–8
oesophageal rupture 37
oncotic pressure of plasma 45
opiates 16, 22, 25, 73
optic neuritis 98
oral contraceptive pill 34, 46
orthopnoea 15
osmolal gap 136, 137
osteoarthritis 113, 114
osteomyelitis 49
oxygen 8, 9, 13

pain
 abdominal pain 51–6
 back pain 114–18
 joint pain or swelling 110–13
 limb pain 49–50
 non-pleuritic chest pain 37–40
 pleuritic chest pain 33–6
palpitation 39, 41–4
pancreatitis 18, 54, 117
panic disorders 44
paraplegia 95, 117
parathyroid hormone (PTH) 152, 154, 155
Parkinson's disease 96
pathological sieve 4
pattern recognition 4
PE *see* pulmonary embolism

pemphigus 129
peptic ulcer 20
pericarditis 33, 35
peripheral neuropathy 91, 93, 95, 96
peritoneal disease 55, 60, 73–5
personal details 1
phobic disorders 44
pinpoint pupils 16
plasma 45
platypnoea 15
pleuritic chest pain 33–6
pneumonia
  abdominal pain 55
  acute respiratory illness 15, 16
  pleuritic chest pain 33, 34, 35
  shock 20, 35
pneumothorax 15, 34, 35, 55
poisoning
  carbon monoxide 88, 89
  food 57
  opiates 16, 22, 25
  strychnine 91
polyarthritis 110
polydipsia 103, 104, 143
polyuria 44, 103, 104, 145, 154
portal hypertension 74, 75, 80
positive predictive value (PPV) 2, 3, 5
posterior fossa 91
post-hypercapnic alkalosis 139
post-renal acute kidney injury 27,
  28–9
post-test probability 2, 3
postural hypotension 88, 89
postural orthostatic tachycardia
  syndrome 44
potassium
  hyperkalaemia 150–1
  hypokalaemia 147–9
PPV (positive predictive value) 2, 3, 5
pregnancy 35, 55, 74
premature closure 5
pre-renal acute kidney injury 27, 28–9
presenting complaint 1
pre-syncope 44
pre-test probability 1, 2, 3, 5
primary polydipsia 103, 104, 105, 143
proctitis 68
prostate 30, 107
proteinuria 46
pseudobulbar palsy 65, 67
pseudohaematuria 107
pseudohyperkalaemia 150, 150–1
pseudohyponatraemia 141, 142
pseudomembranous colitis 68
psoas sign 55
psoriasis 132
PTH see parathyroid hormone
pulmonary embolism (PE)
  acute respiratory illness 15, 16, 17
  information gathering and
    interpretation 2, 3
  pleuritic chest pain 33, 34, 35
  shock 18, 20
pulmonary hypertension 46, 80
pulmonary oedema 8, 15, 20
pulse rate 9, 41, 43, 89
pulsus paradoxus 20
pyrexia of unknown origin (PUO)
  119–23

quadriplegia 117

radiculopathy 91
rashes 54, 129–32

Raynaud's syndrome 49
rectal bleeding 20
renal acute kidney injury 27, 28–9
renin–angiotensin system (RAS) 140
respiratory acid–base disturbances
  133–6, 152
respiratory acidosis 134, 135
respiratory alkalosis 136, 152
respiratory failure 10, 11–12, 13
restrictive cardiomyopathy 80
Resuscitation Council (UK) 7, 8, 41,
  42, 43
reticular activating system 22
retinal artery occlusion 98
retinal detachment 98
rheumatoid arthritis 110, 113
Romberg's test 95
Rovsing's sign 55
ruptured abdominal aortic aneurysm
  51

SBE see standard base excess
sciatica 117
scoliosis 117
'see-saw' breathing 7
seizures 88, 89
sensitivity (Sn) of a test 2, 3
sensory ataxia 95
septic arthritis 110, 113
septic shock 18, 20, 21, 54
serum ascites albumin gradient
  (SAAG) 74
sexual history 68, 107
shingles 54
shock 18–21
shunt 10
SIADH see syndrome of inappropriate
  ADH secretion
sick cell syndrome 141
sideroblastic anaemias 124, 125–6
sinus tachycardia 35, 41, 43, 44
Sjögren's syndrome 110
skin rash 129–32
sleep apnoea 13, 16
smoke inhalation injury 13
Snellen chart 98
'sniffing the morning air' position 7
Sn (sensitivity of a test) 2, 3
social history 1
sodium see hypernatraemia;
  hyponatraemia
somatic pain 33, 51, 54
specificity (Sp) of a test 2, 3
speech 95
spinal cord
  back pain 114, 117
  focal neurological deficit 91, 92, 95,
    96
  frequency of micturition 106
splenomegaly 74, 80, 154
spontaneous bacterial peritonitis 74
Sp (specificity of a test) 2, 3
standard base excess (SBE) 133–4
ST elevation myocardial infarction
  (STEMI) 37
Stevens–Johnson syndrome 129
stiff person syndrome 91
stool 68
straight leg raise test 95, 117
stridor 13, 15, 16, 65
stroke 91, 100
strychnine poisoning 91
subarachnoid haemorrhage 83, 86

swan-neck deformity 113
syncope 44, 88, 89
syndrome of inappropriate ADH
  secretion (SIADH) 140, 141,
  142, 143
systemic causes of coma 23–4
systemic vasculitis 17

tachyarrhythmias 18, 41, 44
tachycardia 20, 44
tachypnoea 20
tension pneumothorax
  acute respiratory illness 15, 16
  critically ill patient 8
  pleuritic chest pain 33, 35
  shock 18, 20
test results 1–3, 5
tetanus 91
tetraplegia 95
thirst 103, 141, 144
thoracocentesis 35
thrombolysis 33, 37, 91
thrombotic thrombocytopaenic
  purpura 30
toxic epidermal necrolysis 129
toxic shock syndrome 129
transient loss of consciousness 88–90
trepopnoea 15
tricuspid regurgitation 75, 80
Trousseau's sign 153
type 1 (hypoxaemic) respiratory failure
  10–12, 15
type 2 (hypercapnic) respiratory failure
  10–13, 15

unconjugated hyperbilirubinaemia
  77, 78–9
unstable angina 37
upper motor neuron lesions 91, 96
upper respiratory tract irritation 39
uraemic flap 57
uraemic pericarditis 30
ureteric colic 117
urethritis 107
urinary tract obstruction 27

vagina 55
'vapid scent' mnemonic 4
vascular claudication 49
vascular disease 23–4, 27, 28–9
vascular dissection 83
venous thromboembolism 46, 49
ventilation 10, 16
ventilation–perfusion mismatch (V/Q
  mismatch) 3, 10, 16, 35
Venturi mask 9, 13, 14
vertigo 101–2
viral encephalitis 22
visceral pain 33, 51, 54
visual loss see acute visual loss
vitamin D
  hypercalcaemia 154, 155
  hypocalcaemia 152, 153
vitreous haemorrhage 98
vomiting see nausea and vomiting
V/Q mismatch see ventilation–
  perfusion mismatch

water deprivation test 105
Wells score 35
wheeze 15, 16
Wilson's disease 80

Z-thumb deformity 113